£3 - 50   15/6/9

G000274797

M.E.

sailing free

NUTRITIONAL ANSWERS TO CHRONIC FATIGUE

Erica White
Dip.I.O.N

i

White Publications ©

First published 1996
by White Publications, 22 Leigh Hall Road,
Leigh-on-Sea, Essex SS9 1RN
© Erica White 1996

Illustrations, cover design: Roydon Hearne

All rights reserved. No part of this publication may be reproduced, stored in a retrieval system, or transmitted, in any form or by any means, electronic, mechanical, photocopying, recording or otherwise, without the prior written permission of the publishers.

British Library Cataloguing-in-Publication Data.

A catalogue record for this book is
available from the British Library.

ISBN 0 9521465 1 7

Printed in Great Britain by
Team Spirit Services

The publishers stress that medical help and diagnosis should be sought before deciding to follow a nutritional regime specifically geared towards M.E.
In addition this book is written in general terms and no responsibility can be accepted for individual situations where self-help is attempted without appropriate professional guidance.

BY THE SAME AUTHOR:

Prices on request from the Publisher:
White Publications ©
22 Leigh Hall Road, Leigh-on-Sea, Essex SS9 1RN
Telephone 01702 72085

BEAT CANDIDA COOKBOOK
A Nutrition Consultant's Collection of Recipes
to use as part of a Four-Point Plan
for attacking Candidiasis.

NOT BREAD ALONE
A Christian Nutritionist looks at Healing and Wholeness

AUDIOTAPES by the author, available from the publisher:

CANDIDA

M.E.

ACKNOWLEDGEMENTS

First, I wish to thank those previous clients of mine who submitted their stories included in Chapter 5: "Now I Feel Great!" They faithfully followed the advice which is outlined in this book, and have been rewarded with success stories to encourage fellow-sufferers from M.E.

I also want to take this opportunity to express my heartfelt thanks to all my family for so lovingly "putting up with Mummy" through all the years when I myself was ill. My fears that the children's memories of childhood would be marred by my constant sickness were unfounded; each one of them has developed into a caring and capable adult, a tremendous example of how all things can be turned to good! My heart is full of gratitude for the warm memories I have of my loving and supportive parents, and my husband, Robin, has never failed to be patient and understanding.

The friends now working with us provide loyal and enthusiastic support; I cannot adequately express the joy of working with a team which prays together! My thanks go to Pat, Pauline, Ann, Frances, Heather and Roger, and also to the ladies who help to shoulder my domestic responsibilities, Lynne and Trish.

I am extremely grateful to Roydon Hearne for taking time from his very busy schedule to design the cover and prepare the layout of this book. However helpful a book might be, its cover has to catch the attention of those who need to read it, in a way which expresses the "feel" of the contents. Roydon has done an excellent job!

Finally, I wish to thank Patrick Holford, not only for agreeing to write the Foreword, but also for making it possible for me to become a Nutrition Consultant by having the vision to set up the Institute for Optimum Nutrition. I was fortunate to have him as my tutor when I trained, and I cannot thank him enough for inspiring me, for passing on some of his enormous enthusiasm and for so obviously having confidence in me.

Thank you, Patrick!

I dedicate this book to Robin -
my partner in marriage, work and life.

CONTENTS

FOREWORD

by Patrick Holford, Founder and Director of the Institute for Optimum Nutrition

Albert Einstein once said, "The problems we have created cannot be solved at the same level of thinking we were at when we created them". So-called M.E. is such a problem and, with old-style medical thinking, sufferers find themselves staggering around in ever-decreasing circles.

I am convinced that the 'chronic fatigue syndrome' known as M.E. is the natural consequence for an individual living in an unnatural environment. By that I mean eating unnatural food, breathing polluted air, drinking polluted water and being exposed to unnaturally high levels of toxic bacteria, viruses and fungi, often as a consequence of an unhealthy digestive tract.

Erica White's excellent book presents a new level of thinking applied to eliminate systematically the most commonly-found contributive factors which lead to M.E. Backed up by volumes of experience, most importantly her own, the information given is highly practical and proven to be effective.

Although necessary to change one's lifestyle, it is never easy but, with good support and management, I am sure that the vast majority of readers will benefit from following this advice and find themselves able to sail free from M.E., back into a way of living which is in line with the natural design of the human body.

Patrick Holford, 1996.

INTRODUCTION

The first two chapters of this book give an overview of my understanding of the way in which the body's immune system becomes overloaded and unable to function efficiently, which I firmly believe should be regarded as the main cause of M.E. rather than placing the blame on a particular virus. "Susceptibility" is the name of the game! These chapters include a discussion of various possible contributing factors.

Chapter Three centres on one of these factors, a yeast called *Candida albicans* which has a great tendency to overgrow in the intestines. An outline is given of the four-point plan which will effectively remove this particular load from the immune system.

Chapter Four looks at a chain of events which can often be seen leading up to M.E., and considers ways in which fear can enter the situation and the importance of understanding the causes of it.

Chapter Five offers brief comments from some of my clients who have successfully recovered from M.E. by following the nutritional approach discussed in the earlier part of the book.

Chapter Six discusses the role of optimum nutrition and the reasons why it is so important in this day and age.

I hope very much that you will enjoy reading Chapter Seven, because it gives an account of my own story of "sickness into health", including my discovery of several of the factors outlined in Chapters One & Two.

INTRODUCTION

These first seven chapters stand alone and would make a book complete in itself on the subject of M.E.. However, Chapter Eight offers an additional discussion for those who are interested in the role of a nutritional approach to health and healing from a Christian viewpoint. For me, this underlies all that I have learned and practise, but I have no desire to force my views on those who do not wish to read them so this chapter forms an entirely separate entity. To those of you who read it, I pray you will be blessed and I guarantee you will be challenged!

At the end of the book you will find practical information on the anti-candida diet together with a suggested menu plan and some sample recipes from my BEAT CANDIDA COOKBOOK[1], also a reading list and other information.

My hope for all who read this book is that you will be encouraged to identify the pieces of baggage which are weighing you down and discover how to throw them overboard so that then you will be able to *SAIL FREE!*

Erica.

M.E.: SAILING FREE

1 No Such Thing?

In the course of my work as a Nutritionist, I often see a client express "shock horror" when I say that in my view there is no such thing as M.E.! However, I quickly reassure them (and hopefully you also!) that I am not in the least suggesting that their symptoms are non-existent and therefore "all in the mind". Far from it! As my own story later in this book will show, I know only too well the pain and misery of long-term sickness, and the frustration that comes from living with constant weakness and exhaustion.

So let me explain what I mean by this rather strong statement. In saying there is no such thing as M.E., I mean that it should not be regarded as one specific illness but rather as a hotchpotch or conglomeration of many different conditions which can vary from one sufferer to another. Researchers around the world all agree that the illness is made up of a combination of interacting factors so that there is no single cause and therefore no single cure.

This means that there are no experts when it comes to dealing with M.E. and the challenge for a practitioner is to discover and identify the specific set of problems affecting each individual sufferer. The most successful practitioners, whether medical or alternative, are those who are the best detectives!

A ragbag of problems

Recognising the illness as a "complex" or ragbag of problems is very important. Let's say that a girl called Mary has been newly-diagnosed by her doctor as suffering from M.E.; if she happens to know someone who has had it and got well, she will obviously want to try the approach which worked for her friend. For example, the friend might have found tremendous benefit from vitamin B or from magnesium injections, but this does not necessarily mean that either of these approaches will be helpful for Mary so that, if her health fails to improve, she will suffer great disappointment and her despondency will increase.

Many who have been formally diagnosed as suffering from M.E. join either the M.E.Association or Action for M.E. in the hope that they will benefit from communication with other sufferers and news of latest research. However, there are many who have never actually received a diagnosis, so they don't even have the comfort of knowing that there are countless others in the same boat; they feel very much on their own, often with little or no support from a puzzled or even sceptical doctor.

Frequently, someone with M.E. is branded a malingerer or hypochondriac, which creates an even heavier burden to bear. In fact, it is estimated that between 100,000 and 150,000 people in Britain alone are suffering from M.E. at any one time.

The illness we are talking about may have as many as sixty symptoms or even more. A client of mine once took the report I had prepared with my findings and recommendations to show to her doctor. In it, I had carefully listed all the various symptoms she had recorded, but the doctor believed they were all a figment of my imagination. The patient carefully explained that the report was based quite factually on the information she had given to me. She really did have a tremendous number of symptoms!

On the opposite page you will see two lists, the first showing symptoms most commonly associated with M.E., and the second being symptoms any or all of which (and more besides!) can occur in any particular case.

Symptoms most commonly associated with M.E.:

- Fatigue not relieved by rest; exhaustion after effort.
- Aches and pains all over, affecting both joints and muscles.
- Dizziness, poor concentration, poor memory, headaches.
- Nausea, wind, bloating, constipation, diarrhoea, irritable bowel.
- Over-reaction to heat or cold - shivering, sweating.
- Mood swings, anxiety, panic, crying, irritability, depression.

Symptoms which may be present:

Muscle pain, muscle weakness, joint pain or swelling and stiffness, fatigue (physical and mental), drowsiness, lethargy, frequent infections of ears/nose/throat, sinusitis, rhinitis, asthma, eczema, acne, itching, sleep disorders, swollen glands, thrush, poor appetite, nausea, wind, bloating, constipation, diarrhoea, irritable bowel syndrome, cravings, water retention, loss of weight, weight gain, headaches, woolly head, lack of concentration, poor memory, anxiety, panic, crying, depression, irritability, mood swings, PMT, shivering, sweating, cystitis, palpitations, visual disturbances, sore eyes, dizziness, numbness, tingling, etc., etc., etc.

Epidemics

Apart from large numbers of isolated sufferers, there have been epidemics where many people have become ill all at the same time, suffering from the same type of symptoms. An early epidemic was recorded in Los Angeles in 1934, where five per cent of the staff in the city's hospitals became ill and stayed ill for several months. Another recorded epidemic was in Iceland in 1948, where five hundred people became ill and half of them remained ill for the next seven years. In England, there was an epidemic in 1955 at the Royal Free Hospital in London where three hundred staff became ill - doctors and nurses - but only twelve patients were affected. It is an interesting fact that this illness frequently afflicts people who are hard workers and therefore likely to suffer from "burnout", typical of hospital staff working very long hours, and it is less likely to afflict those who are resting comfortably in a hospital bed!

What's in a name?

Not surprisingly, some of the names given to this illness are linked with epidemics so that it is sometimes known for instance as "Royal Free Disease", or "Iceland Disease". "Myalgic Encephalomyelitis" actually means, "painful muscles and inflammation of the brain and spinal cord". Although this description might account for some of the symptoms experienced, it does not actually fit many of the great number of varied problems which can be present. These do not all fall within the categories of "painful muscles or symptoms caused by inflammation of the brain". "M.E." is therefore perhaps not the most accurate name which might be chosen to describe this complicated illness.

Similarly, "Post Viral Fatigue Syndrome" is not necessarily an accurate description because in some people there never was a virus, while in others the viral activity still continues, so the illness cannot strictly be named, "*Post Viral* Fatigue Syndrome".

Possibly the most accurate term is the one commonly used in America - "Chronic Fatigue Syndrome" - which gives a clear description of the situation without attempting to attribute it to any particular cause.

One other name which may sometimes be heard, although fortunately not so often in more recent times, is "Yuppie Flu", a title which appears to have started in America because so many young executives were falling ill. It came to be associated with "high flyers" and "over-achievers", but there is nothing in the least accurate about this rather derogatory title because the illness also affects non-executive workers with steady plodding jobs or even those with no job at all!

In Britain, "Post Viral Fatigue Syndrome" is a name which frequently appears in magazines and newspapers but for the purposes of this book I shall keep to the title "M.E.", because this is the name most widely used (if not perfectly understood!) by doctors and sufferers alike.

Possible Causes

So what are the causes of this ragbag of problems? In Chapter Two I shall discuss ten possible contributing factors, many of which are also listed by R. M. Loria, author of COXSACHIEVIRUSES: A GENERAL UPDATE[2], quoted by Doris Jones[3] in the journal, WHAT DOCTORS DON'T TELL YOU in December 1995.

"M.E. is a provocative disease. That is, a range of co-factors - a virus, a viral and a bacterial infection, stress, surgery, vaccination, inherited allergies, toxic chemicals - can make a person susceptible to the virus that appears to cause M.E."

Any of these factors, or others which are mentioned in the following pages, might be overloading your immune system so that it is unable to fight back and allow your body to become well.

2 Possible Contributing Factors

I believe there are at least ten possible conditions which may be major causes of M.E., and it is quite amazing how symptoms of each condition bear a remarkable resemblance to symptoms of the others. What is more, the problems typically associated with M.E. itself could be listed almost identically under each of the ten headings. Each one of the conditions places a heavy load upon the body's immune system, and together they have a cumulative effect which means that immunity becomes less and less effective.

I would like you to imagine that your immune system is a ship - the good ship *"Immunity"*! To start with, *"Immunity"* sails well even though she is carrying a whole lot of cargo. But one day a torpedo hits her and makes a hole in her side, and then the effect of carrying so much cargo on board quickly becomes apparent! The combined weight of the crates and boxes is enough to push the hole below the waterline, so that *"Immunity"* rapidly fills with water and will doubtless sink unless speedy action is taken to identify the heaviest pieces of cargo and throw them overboard. This will lighten the ship and enable the hole to stay above water so that *"Immunity"* stays afloat!

For our purposes, the torpedo might well be a virus or it could be stress or any other factor which is known to damage the immune system. Equally, any of these situations might also be part of the cargo, creating unnecessary loads for the immune system to carry, so we shall look now at various factors which might be responsible. If specific burdens can be identified and removed - thrown overboard - this will enable the immune system to sail healthily on its way, undeterred by minor torpedoes which almost certainly will come its way from time to time!

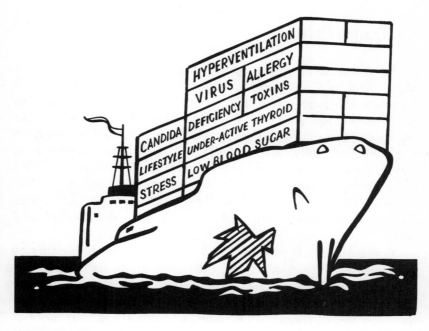

Diagram One: *"Immunity"*

Ten Possible Contributing Factors:

1. Viral infection, past or present.
2. Allergy - food or environmental.
3. Nutritional deficiencies.
4. Toxicity.
5. Lifestyle.
6. Psychological and social factors.
7. Hyperventilation.
8. Underactive thyroid.
9. Low blood sugar.
10. Disturbed intestinal microbes - Candida overgrowth.

Let's take a closer look at these ten points one at a time:

1. VIRAL INFECTION

Several different types of virus have been found in cases of M.E.. One is Coxsachie, of which there are various types all found in the gastro-intestinal tract but with a known tendency to affect muscle tissue. Another is the Epstein-Barr virus which can cause symptoms characteristic of glandular fever and is a member of the herpes family. As you will know if you have ever suffered from cold sores (also caused by herpes), this virus has a habit of lying dormant and flaring up every now and then when the immune system is at a point of extra overload, which might account for the way in which M.E. symptoms sometimes ebb and flow.

Quite often, it is possible to trace the illness back to either of these viruses (in particular to glandular fever) or to influenza or German Measles (rubella) or to a vaccination, even against something which is normally as harmless as rubella. Sometimes the virus is still found to be active, but not always. In normal circumstances, our bodies deal with a virus by bringing into action various parts of the immune system to fight it, so if a viral infection hangs on and doesn't go away, as is often the case in M.E., it is obvious that for some reason the immune system is simply not doing its job. This might be due to one or more of the other pieces of cargo on board the good ship *"Immunity"*. A viral infection could be part of the overload of cargo; equally it might have been the torpedo which made a hole in the side of the ship. Either way, *"Immunity"* is about to go under!

Jane Colby[4], writing in WHAT DOCTORS DON'T TELL YOU in December 1995, says that there is growing evidence which links M.E. to polio. Back in 1948, when scientists first discovered the Coxsachie virus, the symptoms it caused were so similar to those of poliomyelitis that they called it "Atypical polio", a label which was in fact a fore-runner of the names M.E. and Chronic Fatigue Syndrome.

Jane reports that recent advances in technology have placed the Coxsachie virus quite clearly in the polio family tree, and M.E. is now sometimes diagnosed as "non-paralytic polio". Brain scans of M.E. and polio sufferers show very similar marks. The overall similarities of the two conditions are not so surprising if it is realised that the viruses involved are members of the same family and use the same receptor sites in the body's tissues. Before the introduction of polio vaccines in 1954, outbreaks of M.E. occurred immediately after outbreaks of polio in nine out of twelve cases, often involving hospital staff who had been caring for polio patients.

However, Jane Colby goes on to say that unfortunately not all the effects of polio vaccination appear to have been good! Whilst the incidence of actual poliomyelitis fell quite dramatically, it seems to have opened up the way for an increase of other conditions, probably because the eradication of one type of gut virus allows space for others to proliferate.

This seems to be clearly shown by the fact that, in 1959, polio caused eighty-four per cent of paralysis which was associated with an enterovirus (gut bug). As vaccination increased over the next two years, by 1961 the incidence of polio-induced paralysis fell to only twelve per cent, but by that same year Coxsachie viruses were causing as much as seventy-four per cent of paralysis which could be directly associated with an enterovirus.

Yet in spite of these and other facts so clearly set out in WHAT DOCTORS DON'T TELL YOU, there are very many cases of M.E. where no trace of a virus or of viral antibodies has been discovered so it cannot automatically be assumed that a viral infection was a major cause of the illness in these particular instances.

On the other hand, and to confuse the picture even further, it is possible to find people who are carrying Epstein-Barr or Coxsachie viral antibodies but who are not actually suffering from any signs of illness, nor have they ever felt particularly unwell! According to Dr. Thomas Stuttaford of THE TIMES who is quoted by Jane Colby in the article already mentioned, *"...only a small number of those infected with the polio virus became paralysed; about ninety per cent didn't even realise that they had anything more threatening than a cold".*

So what then is the deciding factor as to whether or not someone will develop M.E. or any other virus-related condition? Let me quote a final comment from Jane Colby:

"With polio and M.E., *the state of your immune system governs whether you will be susceptible".* (Italics mine!)

This is an absolute reflection of my own strongly-held belief that a virus itself does not have to be the cause of disease; rather it is the inability of the immune system to fight against it. In other words, if the hole in the side of the ship is already close to the water-line, an added piece of cargo in the form of a virus will ensure that the ship goes down; but if the ship has very little cargo on board, it can cope with an extra unexpected load and still stay afloat!

Leon Chaitow in his book, POST-VIRAL FATIGUE SYNDROME[5] says this:

"There is a viral connection with M.E. in most cases, although we may never be sure whether this is the cause or a consequence of the process. Such ignorance, however, should not stop us from trying to eliminate the continuing viral drain on limited immune resources, while at the same time dealing with anything else which may be further reducing immune competence, such as stress and nutritional imbalances".

So let's go on to look at the other pieces of cargo which might be weighing down the good ship *"Immunity"!*

2. ALLERGY

The term "allergy" is one which is used by different people to mean different things! One argument is that it should be used only in cases of a severe reaction to a substance leading to anaphylactic shock. Some people are affected in this way by peanuts or bee-stings, and they need urgent hospital treatment to reverse the effects and even save their lives.

More commonly, perhaps, "allergy" is used of situations like hayfever or asthma, where pollen or some other factor in the environment causes a reaction in people who have a sensitivity to it. Whether this should correctly be called "allergy" or simply "sensitivity" is irrelevant to the person who is suffering, but "allergy" is the term most often used.

One other situation which frequently goes by this name should probably more correctly be known as "food intolerance". The effects are not so severe that they are life-threatening, but the symptoms can be varied and severely incapacitating, affecting both body and mind in a list which is strongly reminiscent of that list of symptoms commonly associated with M.E.! The difficulty with tracing a food intolerance is that the reactions often occur quite slowly so that it is difficult to discover the culprit food, and the more frequently or regularly the food is eaten, the more "masked" the symptoms become, yet the underlying situation causes increasingly chronic health problems and places a growing burden on the immune system.

For ease of understanding and discussion, I shall follow the common practice of calling each of these situations by the name, "allergy".

It seems that the vast majority of M.E. sufferers have a tendency to food allergies and also frequently react to environmental factors, even though they are often not aware that this situation is responsible for at least some of their symptoms.

The increase in allergy has risen alarmingly in recent years. Official Government figures show that since 1950 children in Britain are six times more likely to develop eczema and three times more likely to develop asthma. The main reason why allergies develop is, once again, that the immune system is not working efficiently. What has happened to cause this situation in less than fifty years?

One factor to consider is that this has been the era of antibiotics. It is assumed that such powerful drugs should enable us to live healthier and stronger lives but instead we seem to develop more and more health problems. It is difficult to think of a single family where at least one member is not struggling with some sort of health problem. Why should this be?

A possible part of the answer is the fact that antibiotics encourage an imbalance of microbes in the intestines, allowing an overgrowth of unfriendly bacteria which among other things cause the intestinal wall to become porous. This leads to the development of food allergies as minute particles of incompletely-digested food leak through into the bloodstream. Also in the last fifty years there has been a general decline in breast-feeding. Bottle-fed babies don't receive the natural immunity they would derive from breast-milk, and in addition they are fed with formulae made from cow's milk which has a very high tendency to cause allergic reactions.

Several other factors have influenced our general immunity over the past few decades. Steroid drugs have become widely used (these include cortisone creams and inhalers, and also the contraceptive pill and hormone replacement therapy, although the women taking them don't generally realise that they are taking steroids!). In addition, immunisation programmes have become the norm and although undeniably vaccines give protection against specific major diseases, at the same time they have a negative overall effect on the strength and efficiency of our immune systems. Also contributing to weakened immunity are the facts that pollution has increased and that there has been a steady decline in the quality of our food; both these situations will be discussed more fully in later sections.

Allergy often "equals" addiction. If you are unknowingly addicted to a food or a drink, possibly tea, coffee, chocolate, alcohol or even wheat or dairy produce - whatever it might be, if a period of time has passed since you last ate or drank it, you begin to get withdrawal symptoms. You will probably not recognise these unpleasant effects for what they are; you just feel a bit "low" or tired or irritable or develop a headache. Because you don't feel too well, you reach for the very thing which you know from experience will give you a "lift" - for a while, at any rate. It might be a cup of tea, or coffee, or a bar of chocolate, or a glass of beer or sherry, or a cigarette - but each time you do this you are "feeding" the addiction. Becoming addicted is a pretty good indicator that you are in fact allergic to the very thing which you feel is doing you good, yet all the time the "lift" it gives is fooling you!

Because the symptoms of food allergy can be so like those of M.E., it is obviously helpful to get them out of the way by attempting to pinpoint and then avoid the culprit food or drink. This will not only considerably improve the overall picture but will also remove a burden from the immune system, a heavy piece of cargo thrown overboard!

Allergy very frequently plays a part in M.E. - sometimes as a major role, sometimes just backstage, but nearly always it is there. It is important to do some detective work to discover just which foods or environmental factors are causing problems, and nutritionists can often help with this process.

The most reliable method for pinpointing a food intolerance also happens to be the most simple and inexpensive! You avoid the suspect food or family of foods for a minimum of five days and then "challenge" by eating it, looking out for obvious symptoms or for a marked change in pulse rate. You need to find a time when you can sit still for an hour (easy if you have M.E.!), and take your resting pulse rate after the first five minutes but before you eat the food. You then eat it and take your pulse again at fifteen minute intervals over the next hour. A change of ten beats per minute either up or down is a significant indication that your body has difficulty in dealing with the food you have put into it. Sometimes the change will be considerably more, sometimes less.

Obviously, you need to avoid the foods which give a clear reaction; those with a smaller change in pulse rate might be tolerated if eaten only at four-day intervals. Sometimes there is no change in pulse rate but obvious symptoms occur, either immediately following the food being eaten or within a few hours. This also is a clear sign that your body would rather not have to cope with it, at least for the time being!

In an attempt to pinpoint environmental factors, I have prepared a questionnaire for my clients which can sometimes be helpful. It might then be possible to avoid the allergen, at least for the time being. Something like a sensitivity to domestic gas can cause extremely unpleasant symptoms as you will read in my story in Chapter Seven, and the answer in that case might be that you have to replace all your gas appliances with electric ones. Regaining lost health can sometimes be a very expensive business!

By avoiding known allergens, you can off-load some cargo so that your good ship *"Immunity"* floats higher on the surface of the sea, and the hole in her side sits more securely above the waterline. Hopefully, later on, when your immune system has become stronger and your ship has sailed a steady course for a while, many of the foods and substances which have previously caused problems will no longer affect you. Sometimes it is helpful to take supplements which will help to heal and restore the intestinal lining so that it is no longer porous.

Meanwhile, some of the symptoms you had associated with M.E. might actually go away if you can manage to discover a previously "hidden" allergy and then take pains to avoid the allergen which causes it.

3. NUTRITIONAL DEFICIENCIES

In the last couple of centuries we have managed to turn our food into substances which contain very few nutrients indeed. In fact, much of what we buy in shops under the guise of "food" hardly deserves the name! Before the Industrial Revolution in nineteenth-century Britain, people did not eat white flour. The invention of steel rollers in mills enabled manufacturers to remove the wheatgerm, the "life", from the grain so that it would keep longer without going bad. The general public liked this new product, believing it to be purer because it was white, and the retailers enjoyed the extra money they made from its longer shelf-life.

Sugar was once a very expensive commodity because it was taxed; when the tax was removed, it became a useful ingredient to include in many foods because of its preservative qualities, and it did not take long for the general public to develop an increasingly sweet tooth, to which food manufacturers were more than happy to pander. At the same time, abattoirs were invented and red meat and animal fat became much more readily available. As the years went on, refrigerators and freezers made frequent meat consumption even more possible. In addition, manufacturers soon realised that chemical additives and preservatives could ensure greater profits, as did farmers using chemical fertilisers and pesticides.

We somehow forgot that food is the fuel for our body's machinery and that, unless the fuel is of sufficiently good quality, the machinery will start to run down and require an increasing amount of servicing, just to keep it going!

Besides having to cope with low-grade fuel, our bodies are infiltrated by an ever-increasing load of pollution from the environment. Small wonder that the machinery sometimes grinds to a premature halt!

Some American research has shown that at least eighty per cent of adults are deficient in one or more major nutrients and that over sixty per cent are deficient in two or more nutrients. The people studied considered themselves to be healthy people. It is safe to assume that people who are not even outwardly healthy will be even more deficient in important nutrients.

What is the purpose of food? Provided it is properly digested, it will be absorbed into the bloodstream as glucose (for energy) but also as vitamins, minerals, essential fatty acids and amino acids. There are many different nutrients in each category and they each have many jobs to do, both alone and in combination with others. Without nutrients we would not be alive!

For instance, protein in the form of amino acids is needed by every cell in the body for all its processes of growth and repair. Consequently, if we are ill, it is vital that we eat good quality protein like poultry, fish, beans and pulses. Essential fatty acids, together with vitamins and minerals, are needed for healthy skin and hearts and strong immune systems, and also to enable hormones to work efficiently. If the nutritional status is good, there is no need for any woman to suffer the monthly miseries of premenstrual tension.

The immune system is made up of many different parts which

all depend on specific vitamins and minerals to do their work efficiently. For instance, T cells and B cells have to be in the correct ratio, and this requires vitamin A, folic acid and iron. Particularly important for the immune system is vitamin C, and our requirement for this vitamin varies from day to day depending on what is happening in the body at any given time. If we are fighting an infection or an allergy, our bodies require far greater levels of vitamin C than when we are well, and it is a useful guide to take vitamin C to what is known as "bowel tolerance" levels. This means that the body will take all the vitamin C it needs and, when it has enough, it will eliminate any surplus via the bowel and cause diarrhoea.

Dr. Robert Cathcart in America has done a great deal of research using very high levels of vitamin C as discussed by Leon Chaitow in POST VIRAL FATIGUE SYNDROME[5]. Twice Nobel prize-winner Linus Pauling was another great enthusiast, as shown by a reported interview with him in the journal OPTIMUM NUTRITION[6] published in Winter, 1994. I have often seen vitamin C taken to bowel tolerance levels be beneficial in turning the tide in chronic illness, and it frequently avoids the need for antibiotics when bacterial infection threatens to take hold.

It is a sad fact that our modern diet, made up as it is of many packaged and prepared foods, contains very little in the way of vitamins and minerals. What is more, drinks like tea and coffee actually deplete the body of vital minerals. In addition, ordinary sugar (sucrose) might be called an "anti-nutrient" for it supplies none of the nutrients required by the body and actually causes a great many problems. More bad news comes from animal fat, which pulls against the benefits of healthy fatty acids found in unrefined oils made from seeds and leads to wide-ranging problems from heart disease to premenstrual tension! Both sugar and fat have weakening effects on the immune system. No wonder our bodies have such an uphill struggle; it is amazing that we ever manage to hold our own against an invading germ! The role of optimum nutrition is absolutely crucial to good health.

4. TOXICITY

Toxicity simply means "the state of being poisoned"! The body needs to defend itself against any form of toxin or poison which appears in the bloodstream, and so in situations of toxicity a tremendous strain is placed upon the resources of the immune system.

Some metals have a toxic effect on the body; these include lead (of which we get large levels from traffic exhaust), cadmium (from traffic but also from factory chimneys and smoke from cigarettes), aluminium (from toothpaste, indigestion tablets, deodorants, saucepans) and mercury (from amalgam fillings in our teeth). Some of these effects are now widely acknowledged. For instance, the British Medical Association has stated that aluminium plays a major part in Alzheimer's Disease or senile dementia, and high lead levels have been shown to cause behaviour problems and learning difficulties in children who live in high risk areas such as London or Birmingham.

Traces of mercury will be found in anyone who has amalgam fillings in their teeth. In Sweden, where it is recognised that mercury is the cause of many problems, it is now forbidden to give amalgam fillings to a pregnant woman because of the possible effects on her unborn baby. In Britain, pregnant mothers are still encouraged to have their fillings free of charge, and you can be sure that most of these will be amalgam. Severe mercury poisoning provokes symptoms exactly like those of Multiple Sclerosis. There is anecdotal evidence that some people have recovered from M.E. when their amalgam fillings have been replaced, but it is very often sufficient to detoxify the body of mercury by taking the correct amounts of appropriate vitamins and minerals, including good levels of selenium. Having the fillings drilled in order to remove them stirs up mercury vapour so that even if a responsible dentist takes precautions to prevent it, an even heavier load is suddenly placed on the immune system which can sometimes lead to a severe set-back.

Traces of toxic metals can be removed from the body by taking a good supplement programme, and the problems associated with toxicity can therefore be largely prevented if action is taken in good time.

Other factors which produce toxicity are the many pollutants in our environment - in the air, earth, rivers, water-supply and sea. There are reports that seals in the North Sea have been dying from viral infections. Viruses have been around for a very long time; no doubt what has changed is the strength of the seals' immune systems which now work less efficiently because their food supply is contaminated with industrial pollutants.

Indoor pollution also has to be recognised - vapour from synthetic materials in carpets and upholstery, insulation, cleaning materials, fumes from domestic gas, etc. Air conditioning makes matters worse by circulating the pollutants. A common phenomenon is known as "sick building syndrome", which means that many people working in a particular building feel ill all the time they are in it, obviously due to environmental factors.

Lack of daylight can be counted as a form of indoor pollution because it leads to feelings of nervousness, exhaustion and irritability. It is important for people with a compromised immune system to receive at least two hours of daylight every day.

Many people are walking around with toxic livers because they have taken so many medical drugs over the years. Residues from these stay with us for a very long time. Then there are those who have a history of drug-taking or of high alcohol consumption, which also leave the body in a toxic state and put a long-term load on the immune system.

Toxins known as "free radicals" are commonly found in food and in the environment as a product of combustion. We inhale them from chimney smoke, log fires, car exhausts or cigarette smoke but we also get them from burnt toast, roasted coffee and the crispy bits on roast potatoes! Seed oils like sunflower oil are extremely good for us if they are not refined and used only cold, but once refined or heated, as when frying chips, they are full of these dangerous molecules called free radicals. They attack us by causing damage to a cell in the body, and the cell, in an attempt to repair itself, takes a bit from its neighbour, thereby causing a chain reaction of damaged cells. Free radical activity is widely held to be implicated in allergy and in many forms of illness including heart disease and cancer.

There is a lot we can do to avoid free radical attack, and obviously it makes sense to do what we can to eat correctly by avoiding cheap oils, etc. It is perhaps even more important to ensure an adequate intake of the antioxidant nutrients which will "defuse" free radical activity - vitamins A, C, E and the mineral selenium, sulphur-containing foods like onions and garlic, and certain amino acids like glutathione and methionine. In nature, oil is always found with its own vitamin E content to help prevent free radical activity. However, the cheaper oils on supermarket shelves have had their vitamin E removed in the "refining" process - no doubt for resale as supplements. We certainly know how to make trouble for ourselves!

5. LIFESTYLE

Our everyday lives often include some pretty negative habits which do us more harm than good. We have already talked about bad eating habits, and how tea and coffee actually block the absorption of many important minerals. Coffee drinkers, for example, are almost certain to be deficient in the mineral chromium because coffee carries it out of the body. There is probably not sufficient chromium in the diet to replace it, and yet chromium is essential for the regulation of the body's sugar stores. Without it, the control of sugar in the blood goes haywire so it is possible that hypoglycaemia or even diabetes might develop, slowly but surely, simply by drinking coffee! Not only this, but the stimulants in coffee and tea are addictive and set up a dependency on them which needs higher and higher levels of stimulants in order to avoid chronic headaches or feelings of jitteriness.

Other addictions, too, place a great strain on the body - alcohol, nicotine, the so-called 'recreational' drugs and also medical drugs like tranquillisers and sleeping pills. None of these do much to encourage the efficient working of our various body systems!

Then there is the question of exercise. The body needs exercise for many reasons, not least because physical movement is the only way we have of mobilising toxins around the lymphatic system so that they can be eliminated from the body via the bloodstream. Lack of exercise means that toxins are likely to stay in us for a lot longer than is helpful, giving rise to feelings of being "out of sorts" even in a normally healthy person.

On the other hand, sufficient relaxation is important for a healthy mind and body. If there is such a thing as an M.E. "type", it could well be a person with lots of "drive" who overworks and is motivated by ambitions of achievement - hence the origin of the title "Yuppie Flu"! To workaholics, sleep is just a necessary nuisance and relaxing with a book or watching television is regarded as an utter waste of time. But the body is designed to need rest at regular intervals, and this is especially important when it has repairs to carry out.

It is good to be determined to beat the illness, and every sufferer should continue to look forward to one day being well but, at the same time, it is important to accept the present situation while it lasts in order to have an inner peace. Frustration and impatience are added stresses, and these alone are sufficient to put a load on the immune system and slow down the healing process. We all need to learn to pace ourselves, even when we are well; when we are ill, rest and relaxation are essential to recovery.

6. STRESS

Both psychological and social factors can have a strong influence on M.E. but sufferers are understandably "up in arms" at any suggestion that their illness is all in the mind.

However, it is an undeniable fact that the immune system is affected by psychological factors such as depression or anxiety or reactions to major life events, and different people have different abilities to cope. This is partly due to previous experience, the way in which we have been "programmed" to respond to situations which have arisen earlier in our lives.

Our ability to cope emotionally also depends on how we are feeling physically. "Stress" is not what goes on "out there" in our lives; it is our inward reaction to those situations. For instance, if we discover a splinter in a finger but otherwise feel quite well, we simply squeeze it out and forget it. But if we are ill in bed with a severe bout of influenza at the time, the splinter can become a source of major anxiety that it might lead to septicaemia, and if we cannot manage to get it out, we remain obsessed with it for hours on end! A vicious circle sets in because a stressful reaction leads to a depressed immune system, and a depressed immune system leads to more sickness and a greater inability to cope, which in turn leads to more anxiety and depression which further lower the immune system, making it less and less able to fight off disease or allergy.

In their book NUTRITIONAL MEDICINE[7], Dr. Stephen Davies and Dr. Alan Stewart state that people undergoing stress are more likely to develop food intolerances and also that allergies are more pronounced when patients are anxious or stressed, but less of a problem when patients are relaxed.

"Social" factors might include any major event which has brought shock or distress. We have to acknowledge that the body is affected by the mind; if you are embarrassed, your face goes red. If you have a shock, your face goes pale and your legs give way. If you are frightened, you get tummy ache and diarrhoea. If you are anxious, you tremble. We cannot deny this strong link between the body and the mind so it is important that everything possible should be done to sort out situations causing worry or depression but, more than that, to overcome negative attitudes towards those situations.

There are many ways in which a nutritionist can give advice to help someone recover from physical and even mental or emotional illness, but some of life's problems will never be solved by nutritional therapy alone! However, a trusting and supportive relationship with a caring practitioner can go a long way towards lightening the stress load. In addition, a carefully-calculated supplement programme which has been tailor-made for a specific individual can do a great deal to improve their stress reactions, which means that they will also find an increased ability to cope.

Whether or not stresses and strains were part of the picture before the onset of M.E., there is no doubt that the illness brings its own overwhelming stress. This needs to be acknowledged and ways found of alleviating the situation as much as possible in order to take the stress load off the immune system. For instance, I have known several people with M.E. who turned the corner towards recovery once they found they could off-load their fears and anxieties on to God, and in their place received faith for the future.

7. HYPERVENTILATION

I include the subject of hyperventilation immediately after stress because people often hyperventilate when they are feeling anxious. Hyperventilation simply means overbreathing, which quickly lowers the level of carbon dioxide in the blood, altering the body's acid/alkali balance and affecting the way our nerves interact with each other. It can lead to muscle ache and fatigue, giddiness, faintness, numbness, loss of consciousness, blurred vision, headaches, nausea, weak limbs, inability to walk, trembling, palpitations, chest pain, fatigue and panic attacks. You can see how this set of symptoms, if experienced continuously, could quite easily be mistaken for M.E.!

Once you have suffered a panic attack in a certain place, perhaps a shopping precinct, the experience becomes associated in your mind with that particular place, so next time you visit those same shops it is not surprising that you feel anxious as you remember what happened the last time you were there, and, because you are anxious, quite possibly you start to hyperventilate. This automatically triggers the physical and mental symptoms of overbreathing, including panic - the very symptoms you were so anxious to avoid! As soon as you recognise what is happening, you need to find somewhere to sit and make yourself breathe deeply, concentrating particularly on breathing out slowly. If you are in a suitable place where you won't feel too conspicuous, it is helpful to breathe into your cupped hands or into a paper bag for a few moments. In this way you re-inhale the carbon dioxide which you just breathed out, and this reverses the symptoms and defuses a panic attack.

Hyperventilation is not always associated with stress; it may simply be due to a habit of shallow breathing or to long-standing tension due to illness, so again there can be a vicious circle. It is important for M.E. sufferers to learn how to breathe deeply and to relax their muscles. Often when we are ill we sit huddled up with folded arms and shoulder muscles tightly clenched. It is a posture which does very little to encourage deep breathing and it is therefore not surprising that symptoms of hyperventilation, so similar to many which we associate with M.E., continue to be experienced.

Frequent or chronic hyperventilation increases stress levels and has the very opposite effect from the inner calm and serenity which it is so important to encourage.

8. INEFFICIENT THYROID FUNCTION

The thyroid is the largest gland in the body. It affects every major organ and stimulates the repair of cells and the manufacture of enzymes. It has a major influence on hormonal function so that an underactive thyroid can lead to problems of menstrual irregularities.

If your doctor orders a blood test to check out your thyroid function, the laboratory technician will be looking for the number of circulating thyroid hormones in the blood sample. However, if you feel cold most of the time, this is a clue that although there might be an adequate number of thyroid hormones swimming around in your blood, they are not actually working very efficiently.

Thyroid efficiency may be tested by taking your underarm

temperature first thing in the morning before you get out of bed. This is based on the work of Dr. Broda Barnes, reported in SOLVED: THE RIDDLE OF ILLNESS by Dr. Stephen Langer and James Scheer[8]. Doing this for two days will give a fair indication but doing it for a longer time would obviously give a more realistic picture. In women, body temperature varies with the menstrual cycle, so it is best to do this test on the second and third days of the period to get the most accurate results. The lowest end of "normal" is 97.8°F or 36.5°C. If the readings are only slightly below this, improvement will often be seen simply by taking a carefully calculated programme of suitable vitamins and minerals. If the readings are considerably lower than normal, some kelp or dulse (seaweed!) supplements in the programme will supply iodine, an important element needed by the thyroid. If temperatures are very low indeed, a supplement may be added which includes the amino acid tyrosine, but this should be undertaken with practitioner guidance.

Normally, with these measures, a slow but steady rise in temperature readings will occur over a few months, indicating an improvement in thyroid efficiency and, almost certainly, at the same time there will be a decrease in many symptoms including chilliness.

In many cases, a low temperature will not necessarily indicate a condition which would be medically diagnosed as an under-active thyroid. We are considering the possibility of what might be called a sub-clinical condition of thyroid inefficiency. Even so, it is helpful to attempt to improve the situation because, once again, many symptoms of an underactive or even inefficient thyroid are the same as those of M.E. - weakened immune system leading to recurrent infections, muscle cramps and pain, aching and stiffness in the joints, intestinal problems of indigestion, gas, bloating, constipation, diarrhoea, etc., poor memory, profound mental fatigue, depression, sore throat, nasal congestion, headache, irritability, etc., etc.

An inefficient thyroid gland makes it extremely difficult to distinguish between the symptoms it is causing and those which might be due to other factors in the M.E. ragbag. Obviously, nutritional steps should be taken to improve the situation if this is indicated by low body temperature, so that at least some of the symptoms in the overall condition may be eliminated or at least improved.

9. LOW BLOOD SUGAR (HYPOGLYCAEMIA)

Imagine a piece of graph paper with a chart drawn across it to indicate levels of sugar in the blood. If you have a chronic condition of low blood sugar, every time you eat some sugar or something which quickly turns to glucose once digested (like white flour or white rice), the level of glucose in your blood will rush to a high point on the graph. If it stayed up there, you would have high blood sugar, or diabetes, so the body very cleverly does something to avoid this happening. The pancreas receives a signal to release some insulin, which allows levels of sugar in the blood to fall by encouraging absorption of the sugar into the body's cells.

However, sugar levels in the blood now drop to a low point on the graph and at this stage your symptoms can be particularly unpleasant. You might feel dizzy and faint, or have a headache, or feel irritable or depressed, or have a panic attack, or just feel plain exhausted.

So, as with an addiction, you reach for something to give you a "lift", something which you have found from experience will pick you up quite quickly. It might be tea or coffee, a biscuit, some chocolate or a glass of beer or sherry! Very soon the symptoms pass and you feel soothed and able to cope once more - but the new-found energy doesn't seem to last for long. This is because your raised sugar level has triggered the release of yet more insulin, so that once again the line on the graph has plummeted down to a low point.

The pancreas starts to over-react and becomes trigger-happy, so the line on the graph goes from high to low to high to low and so on, right across the page! The glands which are trying to control the situation become increasingly exhausted and the situation grows steadily worse. Eventually, the pancreas itself becomes so worn out that it stops producing insulin, so there is nothing to help the sugar level fall, and this is a common cause for late-onset diabetes.

What you need to do is to change the line on your graph from peaks and troughs to a gentle, undulating curve of slight ups and slight downs. You can do this by eating foods which release small amounts of sugar into your blood quite slowly, and by eating at frequent intervals so that you "catch" the line before it drops too low. You also need to take some helpful supplements. For instance, vitamin B3 and the mineral chromium help the liver to release an important substance called Glucose Tolerance Factor, essential to the control of the body's sugar levels. Adequate amounts of the various B vitamins but especially vitamin B5, and also of vitamin C, give support to the adrenal glands while things get back to normal. By improving glucose tolerance, you remove a load from the adrenals and the pancreas so that they no longer suffer from exhaustion and can be restored to healthy function.

In addition to taking supplements, poor glucose tolerance requires an appropriate eating programme, one which avoids foods high in sugar and includes a timetable of eating little and often. The type of food should be chosen for its ability to release energy slowly but surely - good quality proteins like fish, free-range chicken, beans and pulses like lentils and chickpeas, and also plenty of vegetables and whole grains to provide complex carbohydrates.

Low blood sugar gives rise to symptoms which once again are very similar indeed to the those in the M.E. list! What is more, hypoglycaemia can encourage the onset of allergies by exhausting the adrenal glands. Obviously, if glucose tolerance can be improved, many symptoms will be overcome even if there are still more pieces of cargo which are keeping the ship too low in the water! Blood sugar patterns are shown in Diagram Two.

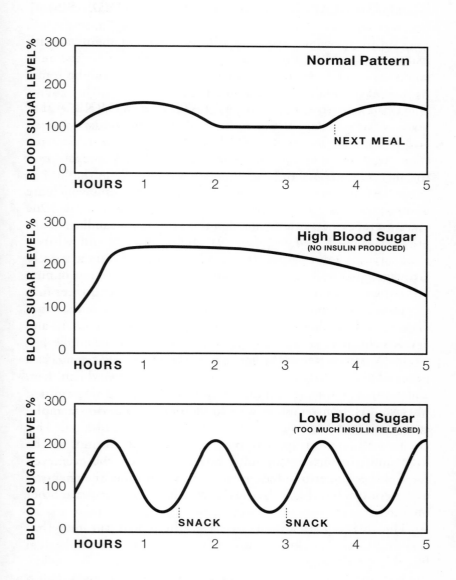

Diagram Two: Blood Sugar Patterns

10. AN IMBALANCE OF GUT FLORA (CANDIDIASIS)

In my experience as a Nutrition Consultant involved with many cases of M.E., this piece of cargo is undoubtedly the most common of all. I would go so far as to say that it can be found without exception in every floundering ship!

Leon Chaitow, in his BEAT FATIGUE WORKBOOK,[9] says, *"What is certain is that concurrent infections such as candida (which very often accompanies M.E.) and hypoglycaemia (low blood sugar) must be considered and dealt with as first priorities if recovery is to be achieved".*

In fact, a severe case of candidiasis has symptoms which are indistinguishable from those of M.E. and the list in Chapter One could be repeated word for word in this section on candida.

The name *Candida albicans* means 'sweet and white', suggesting something delicate and pure. This is a totally erroneous picture because in reality *Candida albicans* is a minute microbe, a yeast, which can afflict us with innumerable symptoms, both physical and mental, many of which mimic other diseases and are therefore frequently misdiagnosed. Its dark and devious character is the very opposite of what its name implies!

Many who suffer at the hands of this microbe see candida as a personal enemy, a dark invader who threatens to overwhelm them and against whom they must engage in long and determined warfare. The only certain way to victory is to understand the enemy's tactics and take the offensive with all guns blazing. This enemy will lose no opportunity to retake lost ground, so the battle must be unrelenting until at last it is won - and even then there is the danger of a false treaty, when you think the enemy is under control but it is in fact just biding its time to make another onslaught!

The imagery of warfare is strengthened by the fact that thriving candida takes on a fungal form, and the ecological function of a fungus is to recycle organic material. To candida, the human body is a pile of organic material and, given half a chance, it will take advantage of a depressed immune system or a deficiency of friendly bacteria in the intestines and start to recycle *us!* Though possibly not a fight to the death, the battle is certainly on for quality of life. Candida multiplies, migrates and releases toxins, causing bowel problems, allergy, hormonal problems, skin complaints, joint and muscle pain, thrush, infections, fatigue and emotional disorders - to name but a few! It is little wonder that candida sufferers frequently say they feel ill all over.

The battle starts in our intestines, where we each carry about four pounds of microbes. When we are healthy, these little organisms are divided into about eighty per cent "good guys" and twenty per cent "bad guys", each with a part to play in our internal ecology. The bad guys are actually quite harmless and even useful while they stay within their "twenty per cent" boundaries, but trouble begins when they overgrow. *Candida albicans* is one of these and unfortunately many things are happening in this day and age which encourage it to grow stronger and to spread.

The situation is largely man-made. Candida is a yeast, and yeasts thrive on sugar, as you will know if you have ever made bread or wine when the process is started by placing sugar and yeast together to "work". In addition to the sugar which is stirred into tea and coffee, it now appears in vast amounts in most commercially-available foods to ensure longer shelf-life and customer-appeal; it is reckoned that modern man eats his own body-weight in sugar every year! Another factor which adds to the body's sugar load is that refined grains like white flour and white rice break down to glucose once digested much more quickly than whole grains, encouraging bad guys to flourish.

At the same time as all this, another situation is causing the good guys to decrease, and that is the indiscriminate use of antibiotics. Many people expect their doctor to prescribe antibiotics for any type of infection, whether it has been caused by bacteria or a virus. In fact, antibiotics are not effective against viruses and, even when used appropriately (for instance, for secondary bacterial infection following a virus infection) these powerful drugs, which so often save lives, not only kill the bug which has caused the illness but destroy beneficial bacteria as well, so that thriving yeasts have more room to spread. Besides antibiotics which are prescribed, we also receive residues of them in meat and dairy products, because many animals are given antibiotics by their breeders purely as a preventative measure to keep them healthy for market.

Another cause of overgrowths of candida is the use of steroids, and this includes the contraceptive pill and hormone treatments which, among others things, suppress the body's immune system. It is fairly common to find young women with severe problems of candida or M.E. who have been on the Pill since the age of thirteen because they had painful periods. It is becoming increasingly common to find older women suffering with similar health problems after being on H.R.T., sometimes for several years but sometimes after only a few months. Seldom has an initial attempt been made to try to improve their menopausal symptoms through nutritional means, yet in the vast majority of cases this is all that would have been needed, and is certainly the best preventative measure against osteoporosis.

People prescribed steroid inhalers for asthma frequently develop thrush infections of the mouth and throat, and steroid creams used for eczema and other skin conditions often lead to problems of weakened immunity. One of the first situations to suffer is the balance of bacteria in the intestines, as the immune system grows too weak to hold back invaders.

Another major reason why so many people are suffering from symptoms related to yeast infection is that we have a generation which to a large extent was not breast-fed, and breast milk ensures that a baby starts life with a healthy balance of friendly intestinal bacteria. It actually contains caprylic acid, an antifungal substance which is otherwise found only in coconuts! The formulae in babies' bottles ensure an early imbalance in the ecology of the intestines.

These and other reasons added together mean that our generation has a problem which is fast becoming epidemic, so it is surprising that many doctors are still not aware of it. Yet in doing research for a dissertation on candida in my third year of training, I found at least one weighty textbook which is probably in most hospital libraries. CANDIDA AND CANDIDOSIS[10], by F.C.Odds, contains well over five thousand medical references to the condition, which means that information on the subject is certainly available to the medical profession.

So what happens when the yeast in our intestines gets out of control? It is actually able to change its shape, becoming rather like mould which grows on an old piece of bread, with little "whiskers" called mycelia that can penetrate through the intestinal walls and invade the bloodstream. In this fungal form, it can travel to any part of the body and establish a colony. It continues to burrow through tissues, ending up absolutely anywhere in the body - perhaps the vagina (causing irritation, soreness or discharge); the urinary tract (causing kidney infections and cystitis); the sinuses, ears, throat or bronchial passages (causing chronic respiratory infections); the skin (causing acne, eczema and psoriasis); the muscles (causing weakness, tremor, numbness, tingling or even paralysis); or the joints (causing stiffness, pain and swelling).

Because the root of yeast infection is in the colon, diarrhoea or constipation (or both!) and abdominal pain are frequently experienced, so that very many people with candidiasis have been diagnosed as having irritable bowel syndrome or colitis. Bloating and wind are very common indeed as the imbalance of bacteria causes fermentation in the intestines. From the colon, the fungus will often travel downwards (causing an itching bottom or painful spasm in the anus); and it will also migrate upwards (causing nausea and pain in the stomach and then soreness and pain of the oesophagus and mouth).

In women, a common effect of candida is to block the efficient working of hormones. This is explained in a practitioners' bulletin I was commissioned to write on candidiasis, available free on request.[11] The other side of the coin is that hormonal changes encourage candida activity, so that symptoms regularly flare up before or after a period and enormous numbers of pregnant women develop thrush. Sometimes, premenstrual or menopausal symptoms are totally due to candida, although usually there are also nutritional deficiencies which need to be corrected. Even infertility can be helped by bringing candida under control and improving nutritional status, and I am happy to have seen several clients, previously infertile, conceive without difficulty when these situations have been tackled.

Once pregnant, it is not a good idea to wage full warfare against candida until after the baby has been born and weaned. This is because dead candida releases a great many toxins into the mother's bloodstream, which obviously does not provide a healthy environment for the baby. However, it is certainly worth keeping to an anti-candida diet during pregnancy and breast-feeding, and also taking a good supplement programme to supply levels of nutrients which not only will help to boost immunity but will also be safe and even beneficial for the baby. With these measures, I have often seen candida symptoms improve during pregnancy, even though candida activity would normally increase at this time. However, as soon as breast-feeding has stopped, it is obviously a good idea to ensure that candida is fully under control by taking all the necessary steps as described in Chapter Three.

Another situation which strongly displays the link between hormones and candida is endometriosis; here again, marked improvements can sometimes be achieved by following the full anti-candida programme.

Men are just as susceptible to candidiasis as women but, partly because candida and female hormones so strongly interact, the symptoms are often more obvious in women. They may have violent mood swings, whereas men are more likely to suffer from persistent depression or bad temper! Women may develop an abnormal menstrual cycle, pre-menstrual tension, periods which are painful or heavy, and countless numbers have chronic vaginal thrush. In men, the most common symptoms are abdominal bloating, wind, and either constipation or diarrhoea, but they also may have aches and pains, depression, anxiety and sensitivities to food and chemicals. It is possible for candida to be transmitted through sexual contact, and so 'thrush' can be passed back and forth between husband and wife.

If a mother is suffering from vaginal thrush at the time of giving birth (which is quite likely to happen because the hormonal changes in pregnancy encourage candida to thrive!), the baby will almost certainly pick it up at the very start of life on his journey through the birth canal. Whilst still inside the womb, a baby's gut is completely sterile. In a healthy state of affairs, the first microbes to enter his intestines will be friendly bacteria supplied in his mother's breast milk. The poor infant whose intestines are populated with unfriendly yeasts even before he has had a chance to suck his first milk is probably going to suffer oral thrush, severe nappy rash and colic in his early weeks and months, and this will quite probably lead to problems of a weakened immune system which in turn will lead to frequent ear infections, tonsillitis and eczema which will then be treated with antibiotics and steroid creams, which will encourage the candida in his intestines to flourish even more! The unhealthy child is all set to become a chronically ill adult.

Someone suffering from candidiasis might as yet have just a few symptoms, or else he might have developed a whole host of different problems. Unfortunately, there is often nothing specific to be seen, and the condition is incredibly difficult to diagnose by any kind of test. Since every person has *some* candida, any test taken will give a positive result, but it seems that many medical practitioners discount this as 'normal', without investigating the level of candida present. Although some types of test are available, there seem to be none which will show conclusively the actual level of candida overgrowth throughout the body or identify satisfactorily its various hiding places (in other words, they are not organ or tissue specific), so very often a person suffering from a whole spectrum of candida-related problems also has to suffer the loneliness of being misdiagnosed and misunderstood and the indignity of being regarded as a hypochondriac. Being told that your pain is 'all in your mind' never helped anyone, and, in any case, where is the help for the mind?

Candida in its fungal form releases a great many poisons (no less than seventy-nine have been identified!) which escape through the leaky gut wall created by candida roots, and among other things they have the effect of causing mental or emotional symptoms - foggy head, feelings of unreality, depression, anxiety, irritability, loss of memory, lack of concentration, inability to make decisions.

Physical symptoms caused by the toxins include lack of energy, weakness, fatigue and muscle ache, which can vary from being slight and occasional right through to being totally incapacitating and seemingly unending.

Added to all this, the body's immune system has such a fight on its hands as it tries to hold back the candida infestation that it is unable to cope with other problems when they occur, and this allows allergies and infections to take hold more easily. It is extremely common to find candida problems in people who have been diagnosed as having M.E. or Chronic Fatigue or Post-Viral Syndrome. This suggests that when a particular virus (causing, for instance, glandular fever or influenza) launched an attack, the body was unable to fight it off because the immune system was already too busy and exhausted from trying to cope with candida. Most of the people I come across had initially been treated with antibiotics, with the outcome that their illness became chronic instead of being simply a short-term attack. I was recently delighted to see in my local surgery a leaflet entitled, ANTIBIOTICS: WHO NEEDS THEM?, an attempt by the medical profession to re-educate the public in their understanding and expectation of antibiotics. Hopefully, the tide has begun to turn.

Food allergy is also very common in candida sufferers. When candida in its fungal form penetrates the intestinal wall, it is thought to make it porous. This means that minute particles of food can get through into the bloodstream before they have been fully digested. In this state, the immune system treats the new arrival as a foe rather than a friend, and it calls out all its troops to deal with it, resulting in a kind of allergic reaction. In future, each time that particular food enters the body, it is recognised by the troops and dealt with in the same way, and we are left with an intolerance or sensitivity to it. An intestinal wall which has become very porous paves the way for a great many "food allergies" in some people, leaving them desperately short of foods they can eat without feeling ill.

Inhaled allergens also become a problem. Things like paint and household cleaners often create a nightmare of symptoms, both physical and mental. Domestic gas and petrol fumes can do the same. Some people experience a horrendous reaction to perfumes or after-shave, which sadly plays havoc with any social life they might still manage to have! Reactions to local anaesthetics have even more dire consequences, as I found to my cost for more than sixteen years.

Obviously, in considering whether to launch an attack against candida, it is important to ensure that the enemy is correctly identified. Before giving nutritional advice, I ensure that my clients have had all the medical tests which their doctors have considered necessary. If no cause for their problems has been found, a suitable questionnaire can then help to ascertain the presence or severity of an overgrowth of candida. For a long time I have used one based on the ideas of Dr. William Crook, who wrote, THE YEAST CONNECTION[12]. If it shows a high score and if doctors have failed to make any other diagnosis, it makes sense to embark on an anti-candida campaign. My own story of lifelong health problems due to candida is written in Chapter Seven of this book, where some of its effects are described from personal experience!

Eventually, after years of sickness, I realised that I had put together a four-point plan which has since been effective in restoring the health of countless other lives besides my own. Later, when I trained at the Institute for Optimum Nutrition in London, I came to understand the biochemical reasons for its effectiveness. In the coming chapter, I give details of this Four-Point Plan.

We cannot put all the blame on candida for ruining our lives; in this day and age we are giving it every encouragement and opportunity to do so. The first stage in fighting back is therefore to start taking personal responsibility for our health.

3 The Anti-Candida Four Point Plan

1) Anti-candida diet.

2) Personal supplement programme.

3) Antifungal supplements.

4) Probiotics - the "good guys".

1. THE ANTI-CANDIDA DIET

The aim of the diet is to starve overgrowths of candida to death! Since sugar encourages and activates yeast, all forms of sugar must be strictly avoided - not just sucrose (packet sugar, whether white or brown), but also lactose (in milk), fructose (in fruit and honey) and malt. Some authors and practitioners allow fruit to be reintroduced after the first few weeks, but I have never seen candida brought *fully* under control whilst any fruit is allowed at all. Refined carbohydrates add to the glucose load so it is essential to use only whole grain wheatflour, rice, corn, etc. Other substances to be avoided are yeast (bread, gravy mixes, spreads), fermented products (alcohol, vinegar), mould (cheese, mushrooms), and stimulants (tea, coffee).

A positive attitude to the diet is essential, and I wrote the BEAT CANDIDA COOKBOOK[1] to show that mealtimes can still be enjoyable! It gives ideas for two weeks' menus together with shopping lists, and the recipes are given a star rating based on the energy required to prepare them! One-star recipes (*) involve little more than opening a tin and a packet, whilst three-star recipes (***) may be served at a dinner party to guests who will be quite unaware that they are eating an anti-candida starter, main course and dessert! The diet guidelines and some sample menus and recipes are included at the end of this book.

A craving for candida's favourite foods is frequently experienced, and at these times steely determination is needed to keep to the diet. However, if temptation threatens to win the day, an amino acid supplement called glutamine can help to damp down a craving for sweet foods or alcohol. Motivation is encouraged by a clear understanding of what is happening. Even when candida-related symptoms have completely disappeared, the diet should be maintained for a further year in order to consolidate the newly-corrected balance of microbes in the intestines, sometimes referred to as the "gut flora".

After being deprived of all forms of sugar for a while, a "sweet tooth" can no longer survive. We were not born with it so, if it is not encouraged, it will go away, making it much easier to stay on a sugar-free diet which of course will help to maintain good health in the future.

It is my fervent hope that the anti-candida diet will be seen as an opportunity to learn how to *enjoy* eating healthily, because this will help to lay a foundation for continued good health in years to come. Hopefully no-one, once cured of yeast infection, will ever again have the slightest desire to eat the type of junk foods and sugar-laden baddies which helped to make them ill in the first place!

2. PERSONAL SUPPLEMENT PROGRAMME

Students at the Institute for Optimum Nutrition learn the basic concept of biochemical individuality and use a Nutrition Programme Questionnaire to assess each person's nutritional needs through an analysis of their symptoms and diet. This simply means that each of us has an individual nutritional status, reflecting strengths and weaknesses of the immune system, etc., which is as unique as our finger-prints, so that we each require levels and balances of vitamins and minerals which are specific to our individual needs.

Buying a pot of vitamins from a health shop might therefore turn out to be a complete waste of money unless the shopkeeper knows a thing or two about the subject and can give you some careful guidance. It is simply not possible for the contents of one particular multivitamin and mineral supplement to meet the exact requirements of every person who buys it!

Our inherited tendencies, medical history, lifestyle and diet all make us biochemical individuals, which means that each person requires a tailor-made programme of supplements which will meet his own specific needs at any given time and so ensure that biochemical and hormonal imbalances are put right and nutritional deficiencies corrected. In this way, all the body systems, including the immune system, may be encouraged to function with the greatest possible efficiency.

A supplement programme of vitamins, minerals, essential fatty acids and sometimes amino acids must be devised to help correct imbalances in glucose tolerance, hormonal status and histamine levels. Appropriate nutrients are also needed to detoxify the body of pollutants, help improve stress reactions and encourage a healthy heart and arteries. In addition, it is obviously extremely important to support the immune system in as many ways as possible in order, among other things, to help it fight back at encroaching colonies of candida. Patrick Holford, in his book, OPTIMUM NUTRITION[13], gives helpful guidelines on how to calculate levels of supplement requirements for yourself; otherwise, a trained Nutritionist will do it for you.

Time and again I have been impressed by the improvement in a client's health when I review their nutritional status after they have been on therapeutic levels of nutrients for a period of three months. This allows time for the nutrients to get into the body and do their work and means that the supplement programme may be pruned down to meet their new optimum level of nutritional requirements. Eventually, it will be cut right down to maintenance levels when this is all that is required to keep their body functioning at its best.

Even this ongoing programme should be tailor-made to take into account specific situations like the presence of mercury in amalgam fillings and, in a post-menopausal woman, the right levels and proportions of nutrients to guard against the possibility of developing brittle bones. This is a far more natural approach than hormone replacement therapy which not only may have hazardous side-effects but almost certainly will depress the immune system, due to its steroid action.

In an otherwise carefully-calculated programme of nutrients, vitamin C may be taken to bowel tolerance levels to rid the body of candida toxins, just as when fighting an infection as discussed in Chapter Two. It is taken at intervals throughout the day until you have a loose bowel motion, and then you stop. Next day, you do the same thing but you will probably find that less vitamin C is needed to achieve the same result. When the body is fighting infection or toxins, its tissues will soak up vitamin C like a sponge, but eventually it will eliminate through the bowel any that is surplus to requirements, hence the loose stools!

3. ANTIFUNGAL SUPPLEMENTS

One of the most useful antifungal agents is caprylic acid, a fatty acid which occurs naturally in coconuts. It is far less toxic than any pharmaceutical antifungal agents, and it has a great advantage in that it does not adversely affect the friendly organisms. Being a fatty acid, it is able to be absorbed through the fatty walls of cells in the body. Taken in the form of calcium magnesium caprylate, it survives digestive processes and is able to reach the colon. For reasons I will discuss in a moment, it is essential to start with a low level and build up slowly.

Certain herbs like oregano, cloves and artemisia produce an oil which also has antifungal properties, and because its chemical structure is smaller than that of caprylic acid, it is even better able to be absorbed through cell walls. This makes it useful for reaching parts of the body where candida has colonised outside the digestive tract, but since the root of an overgrowth of candida is always in the colon, I find that caprylic acid is usually the better supplement to start with, and it might be necessary at a later stage to change to a product with greater systemic activity.

Artemisia, hyssop, golden seal and echinacea are all herbs with broad-spectrum qualities, making them useful against a wide range of undesirable microbes and parasites but with the advantage that they do not disturb the friendly bacteria. This makes them preferable to garlic which, in my experience, is so effective against a wide range of microbes that it also destroys the good guys! A high score on the candida questionnaire together with a history of illness originating in a hot climate are sufficient reasons to suspect the presence of a bad guy other than candida, and to decide to use a broad-spectrum antifungal supplement instead of starting with caprylic acid.

A liquid antifungal substance is available which has a very different approach. It introduces oxygen to the tissues, on the principle that oxygen is antagonistic to yeast organisms. When diluted, it is particularly useful for oral thrush, fungal throat conditions and congested sinuses. It may also be applied to fungal toe-nails!

Propolis is another natural substance which, according to research at the Czechoslovakian University of Bratislava in 1976, is remarkably effective for all fungal infections of the skin and body. It should be taken as an alcohol-free tincture, diluted and increased gradually. Its slightly anaesthetic effect can be most soothing for oral thrush, besides having good antifungal and antibacterial properties. Propolis is made by bees to coat the inside of the hive, which is apparently the most sterile environment to be found in nature!

Aloe vera is gently antifungal and is a refreshing mouthwash or gargle as well as an aid to digestion. It can be used as an overnight denture soak, preferable to products which are not specifically antifungal. Dentures can be an ongoing source of candida re-infection.

Any antifungal substance should be used with caution and special care should be taken when using two at the same time, for instance if you are already taking caprylic acid and then decide to try propolis to help your painful gums. This is because the effect of destroying too much candida too quickly can be quite devastating, as I shall explain shortly.

Tea tree oil is another antifungal substance which, as a cream, may be used for fungal skin conditions like acne, eczema, psoriasis or athlete's foot, and also for vaginal thrush and rectal soreness or irritation. Although skin complaints like eczema are often due to an unsuspected food allergy, they are also frequently fungal in origin and will respond to an anti-candida regime. However, they usually seem to get worse before they get better, as fungal toxins are pushed to the surface of the body!

An effective vaginal cream to use for thrush is one which introduces beneficial bacteria to the tissues and creates an acidic environment to discourage the growth of yeast in the area. This can be most soothing and helpful whilst the four-point plan gets to grips with the internal condition which has triggered the problem. Vaginal thrush will almost certainly not be completely overcome until the balance of bacteria in the intestines has been corrected, but it is great to have help available in the meantime! It is also a good idea for sexual partners to use this type of cream, to reduce the risk of persistent cross-infection.

With careful experimentation, the most suitable antifungal products can soon be found and put to good use, but first you should read the section which follows shortly, headed "Die Off!"

4. PROBIOTICS - THE "GOOD GUYS"

Supplements are needed to carry beneficial bacteria into the intestines and re-establish a healthy colony of gut flora. The Americans call it "re-florestation"! The role of these "good guys" is to increase acidity and to hold back the "bad guys". Tissues densely covered with beneficial organisms provide an effective blocking mechanism against invaders.

Lactobacillus acidophilus is the major coloniser of the small intestine and Bifidobacterium bifidum inhabits the large intestine and vagina. It also produces B vitamins. Other helpful bacteria are Lactobacillus bulgaricus and Streptococcus thermophilus. These friendly bacteria are contained in yoghurt which is therefore helpful provided there is no intolerance to dairy foods. In yoghurt, the lactose content of milk has largely been converted into lactic acid by enzyme-producing bacteria, which accounts for the sharpness of its taste. However, to ensure safe passage of friendly bacteria through the gastric juices, it is necessary to take them in a capsule containing large numbers of good guys freeze-dried in powder form. Two capsules should be taken daily, at breakfast and supper, but may be increased to six daily or even more in cases of diarrhoea or of illness necessitating antibiotics, which further deplete the all-important beneficial bacteria.

Care should be taken that the supplements used contain both L. acidophilus and Bifidobacterium and supply a total of one billion viable cells per daily dose. The product should clearly show its expiry date and the manufacturer should be prepared to supply you with full information. In an independent analysis of twenty-two commercially-available products carried out by the University of Wales, only three came up to specified standards and several brands fell short even of their own stated specifications!

Support

Each of the points in the four-point plan is essential in the fight against candida. Omitting any one of them will end in failure. However, there is also a fifth point which is just as vital, and that is SUPPORT.

Anyone entering the candida war zone will almost certainly find themselves in a minefield of problems. Confusion and depression abound, and someone is needed who can look at the situation objectively, discern what is happening and point the way forward. This is part of the role of an effective Nutritionist.

"Die-Off"!

I have already said that thriving candida releases a minimum of seventy-nine known toxins. Dead candida releases even more. This can lead to symptoms which seem like a flare-up of any of your old problems (for instance, sore throat, thrush, painful joints, eczema) because candida is now dying in the areas where it had colonised, so these are the places where it releases extra toxins and you become aware of the effects.

It can also lead to flu-like symptoms, because large numbers of toxins circulating in the bloodstream can cause aching muscles, fuzzy head, depression, anxiety, irritability and diarrhoea. In fact, they can do almost anything to your tummy, reversing previous bowel habits and increasing nausea, bloating and wind. Perhaps worst of all, they might make you feel severely depressed or anxious.

This unpleasant situation is known as "die-off reaction" (or more formally as "Herxheimer's reaction") and, during these times, you need the courage of your convictions that yeast is actually being brought under control and that you are in fact on the way to getting well!

There is quite a lot that can be done to regulate and control the severity of die-off reaction, but even so you need to know in advance that the going might get rough at times. A large part of my working week is taken up with providing "back-up" support which is offered for three months following each consultation, to encourage my clients to contact me with any questions or problems which might arise.

Die-off needs to be recognised as a last-ditch deception by the enemy because the very presence of the symptoms means that candida is being wiped out and that victory is imminent.

Severe die-off usually indicates that candida is being destroyed faster than the body can eliminate the extra toxins; it can therefore be avoided by reducing antifungal supplements in order to allow the body time to offload the backlog of toxins. The art of the exercise is to destroy candida slowly but surely, and initial die-off will probably be triggered by the diet (as candida is starved to death) and by vitamins and minerals (as they boost the immune system to start fighting back). These first two points of the four-point plan often cause as much die-off reaction as most people want to cope with, so antifungal agents should not be added to the regime until this phase is over.

By the end of a month on the diet and tailor-made supplement programme, the majority of people are able to say that they feel better than they have for years! Then is the time to add caprylic acid or other antifungals together with acidophilus supplements. Sometimes it takes longer than a month for this to be achieved, depending on the situation, but it is certain to come in due course.

Taking ground slowly is still the surest method of attack. Most people on caprylic acid can start by tolerating a medium-strength capsule, 400mg x 1 daily, without too much difficulty. If, after five days, they are not battling with die-off symptoms, the dose may be increased to 400mg x 2, and so on up to six capsules daily. After this, they can transfer to 680mg x 3 and increase again if necessary.

However, the climb up is seldom straightforward as at any stage there might come a surge of die-off reaction necessitating a drop to a lower level, or even a complete break, whilst the body gets rid of toxins. This should not be regarded as a setback, but simply as a necessary part of the process. Drinking plenty of fluid and taking good levels of vitamin C, as already discussed, will speed up detoxification. If a high level of caprylic acid has been taken and it appears to have achieved as much as it can yet some symptoms still persist, it might be necessary to transfer to another type of anti-fungal to finish off the job of bringing bad guys fully under control. Eventually, antifungals complete their work and no more die-off is experienced. The score on the candida questionnaire falls right down to its minimum level, reflecting the fact that the one-time sufferer now feels great!

For some people, die-off reaction is so severe that they seem unable to tolerate even the lowest level of antifungal supplements. This might be due to an already toxic liver, in which case a supplement containing the herb silymarin can help to reduce the toxic load and prepare the way before making another attempt with antifungals. Another possibility is that the immune system is reacting to the toxins released by dead candida; a supplement programme designed to reduce histamine levels will then also reduce symptoms, enabling an easier climb up the antifungal ladder.

Candidiasis is frequently not recognised or even acknowledged by medical practitioners, which means that it is not understood by family and friends. Die-off reaction, even when recognised and regulated by the sufferer, can lead to even more distress when friends and relations expect you to be getting better yet you are actually feeling and looking worse. Loneliness and despair add to the physical and mental suffering created by the enemy within. It is a scenario well-known to M.E. sufferers.

Problems along the way

Occasionally, little or no progress seems to be made in the candida battle. When this is the case, there is always a reason which needs to be found. It might be that some other piece of unsuspected cargo is putting a load on the good ship *"Immunity"*, something like food intolerance or amalgam fillings in the teeth. Amalgam contains mercury which is a toxic metal. Its continual presence in the body requires the immune system to work extra hard. If nutritional steps to detoxify the body seem unable to cope with the situation, it is sometimes necessary to have amalgam replaced by less toxic fillings.

Sometimes little improvement is seen because the digestive system is not effectively breaking down food into nutrients which can be absorbed into the bloodstream, and so the immune system is not receiving the boost it requires. This can even mean that food supplement tablets pass straight through and out the other end, in which case they have obviously had no opportunity to do their work! If this problem is identified, it can be helped by taking digestive enzymes and possibly hydrochloric acid supplements for a while to boost the gastric juices.

A hold-up might be due to environmental reasons. It is sad but true that your home could be making you ill. The house should be inspected for any damp or mouldy places, especially in the kitchen or bathroom but also round the frames of double-glazed windows, which need to be regularly wiped with an antifungal preparation. If you own some house-plants, the very air you breathe as you sit in your living-room will be full of air-borne spores rising from mould in the soil. You really need to find good foster-homes for your treasured plants and in their place, for Christmas and birthday presents, ask for some of the beautiful silk arrangements which are available now. It is amazing how often my clients do not take this caution seriously, because we are as sentimental about our plants as we are about our pets! The fact remains that it is likely to make an enormous difference to how ill or well you feel, because a candida-sensitive immune system will react to any of its yeasty relations, including mould.

The area in which you live might also play a part. Several people have told me that their illness began after they went to work in an oil refinery, or even to live close to one, and chemical smells carried by a prevailing wind can sometimes lead to a definite worsening of symptoms. Even in the country, pesticide sprays put a tremendous load on the immune system triggering asthma and other complications, and vast fields of rape seed in bloom ensure a difficult few weeks each summer for a great many people. In Autumn, rotting leaves can lead to a worsening of symptoms for many yeasty people, and a holiday in Northumberland was once ruined for me by visiting a musty castle!

Just occasionally, it has to be said, I discover that some-one is not getting well simply because they are not being strict with the diet! Friends and relations persuade them to have a piece of Christmas cake, or some raspberries from the garden, or a glass of wine at a birthday dinner, and people are very good at saying things like, "It can't *possibly* make any difference! Everyone knows that fruit is *good* for you! Anyway, who says this diet is going to help you? Nothing has actually been *proved*, has it? You can always go back on the diet tomorrow, if you *really* think it's doing any good, but *I* think you've lost an *awful* lot of weight. It *can't* be good for you!"

It is absolutely essential to be totally motivated to sticking to the diet and to have the courage of your convictions in order to withstand such pressures from your nearest and dearest. Not to do so is a waste of your time and money and will certainly slow down the speed of your recovery. What's more, it will lead to another bout of die-off to live through - and you are the one who will have to endure it, not your sceptical mother-in-law!

Slow progress might be due to environmental factors (for instance, domestic gas or mould from house-plant soil) or food sensitivities over-loading the immune system. Avoidance of culprit foods once identified through pulse-testing (see Chapter Two: Allergy) not only removes some symptoms but also removes a load from the immune system, enabling it to work more efficiently. Very often, once candida is under control, porous intestines can be helped to heal by taking butyric acid or other helpful supplements and, after a while, the foods may often be re-introduced without problem.

Discovering environmental culprits is possibly more difficult and involves detective work. As already mentioned, it might also incur considerable expense if, for instance, a reaction to household gas is discovered and you have to buy an electric cooker and heating system, as we once did! The improvements in my health made it very worth-while and several years later we were able to have a gas boiler re-installed, together with beautiful gas-flame fires!

The way ahead

There is no easy way to win the candida war. It takes courage, determination and perseverance - but it can be done. For more than fifty years I fought an unidentified foe. In my own experience, the unmasking of the enemy was the initial breakthrough; the four-point plan brought victory, as you can read in Chapter Seven.

You know that candida is under control when you are free of symptoms; it's as simple as that! It's a good idea to check your score on the candida questionnaire, to make sure it has reached its minimum level.

It is then wise to experiment cautiously with relaxing the anti-candida diet for a month, to see if this will cause a return of any of your old symptoms. I usually suggest a small amount of wholemeal yeasted bread, some crisp fruit (apple, pear), low-fat milk and some Edam or Gouda cheese, unless there is a known intolerance to dairy produce. It is sensible to continue taking antifungal supplements and acidophilus during this month to provide some "cover" if the experiment turns out to be a little too early and symptoms start to recur, in which case you need to return to the diet for a month or two longer and then try to relax it again.

However, if all goes well with the experiment, it is then safe to stop taking antifungals and acidophilus supplements but important to continue on a maintenance programme of vitamins and minerals to keep your immunity boosted. It is also necessary to return to the diet for a further year in order to consolidate the newly-established healthy balance of bacteria which will just have been achieved in your intestines. You have a little more leeway than before to break the diet (sensibly!) if you are eating away from home on the odd occasion, but to do so every day would re-activate the candida before the good guys had had sufficient time to be strongly re-established.

Exercising self-control and patience in this way is well worth while because, at the end of the year, you will almost certainly find that you can transfer to a general healthy diet which includes wholemeal yeasted bread, fruit, cheese and a little alcohol. As a Nutritionist, I feel I have failed in my job if my clients have the slightest desire to return to sugar or junk foods, because the anti-candida regime is an excellent opportunity to learn how to enjoy eating all the healthy foods which are available to us, and there is no point at all in returning to the type of food which helped to make you ill in the first place!

I believe there is less chance of candida being reactivated in someone who has brought it under control and has also boosted their immune system to keep it that way than there is of someone experiencing its symptoms for the very first time. The difference is that someone who has recovered knows how to avoid a recurrence, whereas the person who has just developed thrush or rectal irritation usually has no idea that it is being caused by his or her diet and lifestyle! Who, knowingly, would choose to walk back into trouble?

4 A Chain of Events

You have just read a discussion of what I regard as the ten main possible contributing factors in M.E., and I have given by far the largest space to candida. This is because, of all the possible pieces of cargo which weigh down the good ship "*Immunity*", candida is without doubt one of the heaviest and most frequently found, usually stowed down in the hold where it has been travelling undetected!

Candida has certainly been a factor in every single case of M.E. which I have come across, to a greater or lesser extent - usually greater. It is therefore vital to do everything possible to ensure that an overgrowth of candida is brought totally under control, and this will not be achieved unless it is attacked with all guns blazing. Omitting just one part of the four-point plan, or failing to keep strictly to the diet, is certainly sufficient cause to lose the battle.

In its role of weakening the immune system, candida can be seen as taking its place in a chain of events frequently found in the history of an M.E. sufferer. This chain of events is listed opposite.

It would not be true to say that the cumulative effect of previous situations is always the case in M.E., because sometimes a sufferer has fallen prey to a virus which has hit him seemingly out of the blue. However, M.E. does very often set in after a gradual build-up of events, and getting to the root of the problem is like taking layers off an onion as each successive situation is discovered and dealt with in turn. As I have tried to make clear, I strongly believe that the key to the cure of M.E. lies in realising that the main cause is not an invading virus but a person's susceptibility to that virus. A bug which threatens to overwhelm your immune system can only do as much harm as your immune system will allow it to!

Frequent Chain of Events:

- Minor health problems over many years with frequent antibiotics and/or the Pill,
  leading to ...

- Yeast in the intestines spreading and becoming fungal,
  leading to ...

- Digestive symptoms, general tiredness, sugar craving,
  leading to ...

- Acne and other skin problems, often more antibiotics or steroid creams,
  leading to ...

- Allergies, cystitis, thrush, menstrual problems and PMS, often hormone treatment or more steroids,
  leading to ...

- Extreme tiredness, mood changes, irritability, poor concentration, poor memory, anxiety, depression, migraines, insomnia, lack of appetite,
  leading to ...

- Severe immune suppression, extreme susceptibility to infection, multiple allergies, chronic fatigue.

An effective immune system would allow no house-room to an invading virus; the attempted attack would be thwarted, the virus would be controlled and ill-health would be avoided. The answer therefore is to reduce susceptibility. This can be done through taking the following steps:

1. Making changes in lifestyle and eating habits.
2. Correcting the balance of bacteria in the intestines.
3. Boosting the immune system and nutritional status with adequate supplementation.
4. Removing all identifiable loads from the immune system.

In these ways, the body can become strong enough to fight back and destroy any invader which has been able to penetrate its defences, whether it is a virus, fungus, allergen or some type of bacterial infection.

A Nutritionist can help to unravel the complicated tangle of events and situations which together have caused M.E., but in the final analysis the responsibility for healing and for health lies with only one person - the sufferer! Some folk are just not prepared to do what it takes. They cannot really believe that the food they eat has anything to do with their state of health and they will not countenance the idea of giving up tea or coffee or chocolate or anything else which might be having adverse effects on their bodies, even on a trial basis to see if it helps. They believe I am trying to deprive them of one of the only pleasures in life which they are still able to enjoy. This is understandable and of course they are free to choose, but they really need to consider that eating gives only a momentary pleasure, whereas the joy that comes with a healthy body will last for years!

Others may be willing to make drastic changes to their eating habits but there might still be stressful circumstances in their lives which are placing such a load on their immune systems that no amount of good nutritional advice will be able to restore their health! As already discussed, it is really important to find ways of dealing with stress, either by taking steps to sort out the underlying problems or else by finding ways of alleviating its effects or even of rising above it!

I cannot leave a consideration of the emotional aspects of M.E. without mentioning fear. It is not in the least surprising that someone with M.E. should be full of anxiety about his health and his future, for so many aspects of life are affected - relationships, finances and career prospects, at the very least.

One way in which fear takes hold is over the question of exercise or activity. Many times I have seen someone who is recovering well, and then one day they ring me to say, *"I overdid it yesterday, and I feel as though I have put myself back to square one. I won't do that again in a hurry!"*.

A fear was implanted way back in their illness that M.E. gets worse if you do too much, and now they have just proved it to themselves by spending a lovely day walking, only to be full of aches and nausea and exhaustion the very next day. Something needs to be explained.

Since candida is invariably part of the problem, their strengthening immune system has been busy bringing yeasts under control and this means that a large number of toxins will have accumulated in the body. These toxins collect first of all in the lymphatic system, which needs to empty its contents into the bloodstream via the thorax, at the base of the neck. Once in the bloodstream, these toxins make their presence felt by causing aches and pains, headaches, nausea, diarrhoea, depression, and so on - all the typical symptoms of die-off reaction. However, this is an unavoidable part of the process of detoxification, because toxins need to enter the blood so that, when it is filtered by the kidneys, the toxic waste products can be eliminated from the body in the flow of urine. The problem is that, unlike the circulating bloodstream which is pushed around the body by the heart, the lymphatic system has no pump, and it is only the physical movement of our muscles which sends the toxic contents of the lymphatic system on their way to the thorax to be tipped into the bloodstream!

In other words, the unpleasant symptoms experienced after exercise or activity are in fact a very good thing because it means that in a day or two you will feel several degrees better than you did before! Of course, the amount of activity needs to be monitored so that the stirred-up toxins do not lead to too many unpleasant symptoms, but basically you need to realise that a certain amount of exercise is beneficial and will speed up the rate at which your body can offload the toxins which are being produced by dead candida.

Even someone who is very ill and bed-bound is well advised to do gentle assisted movements of arms and legs to aid in this process, and should not be afraid to do so.

For someone who has already made a big break-through in health and is almost completely well, it is obviously most distressing to suddenly feel that they have taken a backward step. I well remember the lady who told me that she had been Scottish dancing for the first time in eight years, a joy she thought she would never again experience! Her delight knew no bounds - until the next day when she rang again to say how ill she felt and was afraid she had overdone it and brought it on herself. I was able to reassure her that no doubt her lymphatic system had been working overtime due to all the unaccustomed activity of her muscles, and that almost certainly in a few days' time she would be feeling better than ever. She was!

Another aspect of fear is that it often seems to have become an integral part of the illness, so that eventually the sufferer is even afraid of becoming well again. After months and years of chronic illness, the possibility of a healthy future is often regarded not only with incredulity but also with a fair amount of trepidation.

In addition, I often find people who are afraid to admit that they are now completely well, even when they very obviously are! Sure enough, they had suffered from M.E. for a long period of time, but now they are back at work and coping with home and family, experiencing no more tiredness at the end of a busy day than any other normally busy person.

Yet they still hold on to the identity they have known for so long, still think of themselves as "having M.E." If they approach me for a review consultation, being determined to stick to a good nutritional programme in the future, they still write on their questionnaire that they suffer from M.E.!

My job then is to assure them that no, they do not! They need to be encouraged to recognise and come to terms with how well they have become. It is a sort of identity crisis, and for some it can take a long time before they are ready to admit that they used to have M.E., but that now they are well!

Sometimes I am asked to get involved at this level by praying that they will be set free from the fear that grips them. Other times I hear from an ex-client that they have realised for themselves how fearful they had become and, as a consequence, how much it had held them back from experiencing the joy that *should* have been theirs when their health and strength were restored. Having made the realisation, they have then made a determined effort to break free from the bondage of fear, with happy results!

It is a common occurrence, and one which I feel needs recognition and help more than is generally realised.

But people *do* break free and they *do* become completely well! If you feel doubtful about this, the next chapter should help to convince you!

5 *"Now I Feel Great"*

For someone starting out on a nutritional regime, the road ahead can seem long and uncertain. Recommended changes in diet may be radical, affecting family and social life, and the cost of supplements reaching on into an indefinite future can be daunting, involving sacrifice and financial planning. Does the programme really have to be so strict and so demanding? In the end, is it really going to prove worthwhile?

If you are in the process of weighing up the possible pros and the undoubted cons, or if you simply need assurance that the nutritional advice you have decided to follow really is likely to bring some benefits, I suggest that you read the following accounts collected from several of my clients who, like you, had to adjust to a new way of eating, find money for supplements and consultations, frequently coping with die-off reaction from candida toxins and withdrawal symptoms from caffeine, and all the time wondering whether this really was the right thing to do and whether, in due course, they would actually reap some benefits!

I feel certain you will be encouraged and who knows? *Your* name might well be one of those appearing in my next collection of testimonies!

CLIVE, a young man from Essex, had been diagnosed by his doctor as suffering from M.E. eight years previously, at the age of nineteen. He describes himself as going from happy and fit to being depressive, ache-ridden and permanently tired. On doctor's advice he took anti-depressants and gave up sport. He says:

"*These things didn't seem to make any difference and my life took a downhill turn. I stayed feeling dreadful for about three years during which time I had to give up a university course.*

For some unknown reason I gradually started to feel a little better but was still feeling worse rather than better for most of the time and needed large amounts of sleep. After a further five years of being very up and down I met Erica while servicing her computer! I started on the anti-candida diet which seemed very daunting at first but I was determined to get myself fully fit again.

After the first three months I was starting to feel a bit better but not great. The die-off reaction of the antifungals was hard to handle because just as I was starting to feel better it would knock me down again. Fortunately with time these bouts got less frequent which made things easier.

After a year on the diet I tried relaxing it for a month and had no side-effects so gave up the antifungal supplements. Going back on the diet for a further year, as Erica advises, has been no problem because I have found that I now prefer soya milk and soda bread to their 'yeasty' equivalents.

I feel confident that I have kicked my M.E./Candida problems and am feeling fully fit for the first time in eight years. I can go to bed late and get up early without suffering the next day. Standing up and concentrating for long periods causes no problems and I can now say that I feel content with my life and don't worry much at all. It is great to feel so fit again after such a long time."

ELISE, from Aberystwyth, had suffered from M.E. for eight years but also from other health problems all her life. She writes:

"*Two and a half years ago, after having my baby, I simply didn't get better. I'd eaten anything and everything during the pregnancy, and felt well at the time even though I know now that I had probably suffered seriously with candida since eight years ago, which was when M.E. set in. Out of desperation I contacted Erica and started immediately on the diet and vitamins and minerals she advised, adding caprylic acid (to kill yeast) and acidophilus supplements (to restore the friendly bacteria) a month later. Post-natal depression was severe for three months; belching, little appetite and fatigue due to die-off were severe, compounded by little sleep. Erica's supplements dealt with the post-natal depression also, so that within eight months I felt almost normal, but with not much energy. Although die-off was severe, at least I could control it by the dosage of antifungals and vitamin C intake. My lifelong problems started to disappear - after 'flaring-up' quite badly - such as cystitis and thrush, and by the first summer I was well, although still very tired.*

Last summer I started to play badminton and was pleased with my level of fitness - the first time to have been fit in fifteen years! It takes a long time, but perseverance pays off when you have help to know what you're doing."

JILL, from Swansea, had been medically diagnosed as having M.E. for more than two years. After she had followed my advice, I was thrilled to receive this letter:

"Just a few lines to say many thanks for all your help and support since I started treatment for candida.

Before starting treatment I had been diagnosed M.E. (of unknown cause - no virus was found) and had become so ill that I was bed-bound and house-bound for two years.

Before my illness I was an NHS Senior Physiotherapist and played a lot of sport, tennis and squash to a very high standard. I was amazed that the medical profession couldn't help me - all I was told was "rest"!!

In my prayers I asked God to give me a sign if he was able to help me. Within days I saw your "Beat Candida Cookbook" advertised and after reading it I knew what was wrong with me! I started on a candida regime and slowly but surely I started to improve. I knew I was on the right track!!

During the times I felt discouraged along the way, you were always there with encouragement, help, support and enthusiasm. Your personal approach is invaluable to me and your other clients.

After six months of treatment, I have more energy, my head is clearing and my brain is working properly again! I can walk further and have started driving again short distances, also gentle swimming once a week. My quality of life has improved beyond recognition - it's wonderful!!

All my friends and family are amazed at my improvement. Every day I thank God."

DEBBIE, from Hampshire, had been diagnosed as suffering from Post Viral Fatigue Syndrome nineteen months before she contacted me. Eleven months later, she wrote:

"I feel like a new person! I am able to tackle mowing the lawn and other household tasks without collapsing in a heap for days afterwards. The improvement in my health and energy has been so remarkable that I don't regret embarking on this diet at all. A positive outlook, determination and an iron will are all that is needed!"

When FIONA, from Essex, first contacted me, she had been diagnosed with Chronic Post Viral Fatigue Syndrome seven months previously, and was consulting a Neurologist who had prescribed antidepressants. She had been too ill to continue her first year at university but, having first consulted me in January, she was fully fit and able to resume her studies in the Autumn term. She wrote her story for this book during the Christmas holidays, having successfully completed a full and happy term!

"Having collapsed in a university lecture, I was told I would be ill for about two weeks. I waited with great frustration, only to find that three months later I still could not even walk. I had no memory or concentration. Despite feeling exhausted, I could never sleep until the early hours of the morning, and then would wake feeling as though I had run a marathon! I could not cope with light, noise or conversation. I had so many blood tests, the nurses joked that I might 'dry up'!

In pain and bed-ridden, I wondered what was happening to my body. Glandular fever was then diagnosed, but a few months later I was feeling even weaker. I struggled to get back to university but only managed two lectures in a whole term. I couldn't manage stairs

*and when I first went to the supermarket I just wanted to lie down
in the middle of the aisle. My muscles still ached, especially when I
used them!*

*Finally, I saw a Neurologist who gave me a brain scan and told
me I had a classic case of M.E. He confirmed that my brain did
actually exist but that it was working like a 'faulty computer
programme'!*

*The university tried to encourage me to take a year out to
recover. I eventually gave in and later discovered Erica's nutritional
regime with the anti-candida diet. My headaches immediately
disappeared; I had forgotten what life was like without them. From
then on, my symptoms gradually left.*

*I am now relaxing the diet, having been on it for a year, and
have completed a term back at university (including a game of
hockey and an all-night Ball!). Friends are amazed at the speed of
my recovery and it feels so good to have my health back. I have been
challenged by the amount of sugar I was consuming. The diet has
been the key to my recovery (along with the prayers of many
friends). I have been really blessed and supported by Erica and her
staff, and my eyes have been opened to the basic fact that what we eat
will hugely affect our health and general well-being."*

In compiling this little collection of encouraging experiences I
have to give pride of place to the following, because it is written
by a lady aged ninety-one who had suffered for several years with
chronic fatigue, sinusitis, thrush and gout. ELIZABETH, from
Kent, writes:

*"When I started work with you a year ago, I was on the eve of
my ninetieth birthday. I count this as an advantage because it made
me realise that I may not have very much time left for
experimenting, and if relief from candidiasis can be achieved at this
age, there is hope for a lot of other elderly people who may think they
are too old to do anything about their own problems.*

*When I started I also had another advantage. I was already a
convinced believer that optimum nutrition could and would act as a
healing agent and I brought to your programme of treatment a*

feeling that if I kept to the regime for long enough and strictly enough, I should automatically get some relief, even if not a complete cure. Fortunately, I live alone and so can eat what and when I like, and this, again, is a great advantage for anyone starting such treatment.

For a number of years before beginning work with you, I had had very painful feet, which greatly hindered my walking. Also, I had become completely deaf, so much so that I could hear nothing at all. It felt like being in prison and out of the world. I also suffered from what is now known as chronic fatigue syndrome. I was so tired all the time that I had to force myself to do even the simplest and most necessary things to keep going.

And now, after a year's faithful adherence to all your suggestions and recommendations, I feel a completely different person. The gout in my feet has completely gone; the catarrh in my ear, which had prevented me from hearing, is definitely clearing up, and I no longer wear a hearing aid as my hearing has improved so much. I am beginning to catch up with all the jobs I should have done long ago in my capacity as manager of a block of thirty-two flats. I also do all my own shopping and cooking and all the other things necessary to keep alive."

Is further comment needed?

6 The Importance of Optimum Nutrition

Almost every family today has at least one member who is suffering from health problems of some sort, often of a mysterious and unaccountable nature. Many people react to various foods and chemicals, and some are allergic to almost everything. Our immune systems are finding it increasingly difficult to cope under the strain of all that is being thrown at them; our bodies were not designed to run on refined grains, added chemicals and polluted air.

It has been estimated that in one year the average person inhales two grams of solid pollution from the air, eats twelve pounds of food additives and consumes one gallon of pesticides in fruit and vegetables. We also take in nitrates from water and hormones and antibiotics from animal produce. This is all in addition to the problems caused by our high sugar, high fat, refined grain diet!

The industrial revolution of the nineteenth century introduced many blessings to our civilisation, but it also led to catastrophe in terms of our food. New steel rollers in flour-mills brought white flour - and white bread - into our lives, with longer shelf-life to satisfy the retailers, but less fibre to keep our intestines healthy. To the consumer, white flour seemed purer than wholemeal, and it soon became the basis of our diet. At about the same time, the tax on sugar was lifted. Since sugar acts as a preservative, manufacturers began to include it in as many products as possible - and this country now leads the world in its production of cakes and biscuits made with white flour and sugar.

Abattoirs were invented so that animals were slaughtered on a vast scale, and for the first time in history we could eat meat three times a day - bacon or sausages for breakfast, ham or luncheon meats at mid-day, and meat or meat-products like burgers for dinner. Our intake of saturated fats soared - and so did heart disease, which was previously quite rare.

In the first world war, hydrogenation was developed. This process turns oils into spreadable margarines, and for the first time there was an alternative to butter or animal "dripping". The consumption of margarine trebled in five years - and the incidence of heart disease rose even more. The reason for this is that hydrogenation turns 'cis' fatty acids in natural unsaturated oils from seeds into 'trans' fatty acids, which have even more harmful effects than saturated fats from animal products. The chemical structures of the different types of fats show this quite clearly, but the consumer is generally not aware of the situation. (Next time you buy margarine that claims to be high in polyunsaturates, look for the small print to see if it states 'hydrogenated'. If it does, put back the tub and look for one of the few which claim to be *unhydrogenated* - in other words, solidified by the less harmful process of emulsification.)

In the first half of this century, our diet changed from being mainly vegetables and starch to containing as much as sixty per cent fats and sugars. We also changed to a more sedentary life-style; we started to drive to work, sit down at desks all day, spend the evenings listening to the radio or watching television, and buying our food in tins and packets instead of digging up the garden to grow it! We created a totally artificial energy balance, and our level of fitness deteriorated as a result.

As Third World countries latch on to 'civilised' habits, their populations not only continue to suffer from deficiency diseases but also, increasingly, from our Western diseases. Problems like heart disease and diabetes, once comparatively rare, now afflict the more Westernised sections of under-developed countries as much as our own. The situation is spreading.

Yet most of us consider that our dietary habits are 'normal'. If the truth be told, in the last couple of centuries we have completely forgotten what a 'normal' diet should be!

The majority of people are ignorant of what is happening.

Like me a few years back, they have no idea of the connection between food and health. It is interesting how many of these same people insist on four-star petrol for their cars! However, public awareness is increasing, and environmental issues form a growing part of political policies. It is becoming more generally known that lead from car exhaust can affect children's brains, causing learning and behavioural problems. People are beginning to suspect that they might feel better than they do if they knew more about which foods were good for them. Migraines are commonly accepted to be triggered by chocolate, cheese or coffee. The British Medical Association recently announced that aluminium has been found to play a major role in Alzheimer's disease - senile dementia.

But who is telling the public where the aluminium comes from? Do they know that it's not only in their pots and pans but also in their indigestion remedies and deodorants?

Do they know that even lead-free car exhaust is dangerous because of the free radicals it carries? (See Chapter Two: Toxicity) Do they know that free radicals are also rampant in many oils when heated so that the only really safe way to fry or to roast is in extra virgin olive oil? (Polyunsaturated oils like sunflower seed and safflower seed are excellent for health when used cold in salad dressings and should be eaten daily, but they produce a large number of free radicals when heated to high temperatures.)

Do they know, in addition, that using refined white flour instead of the whole grain alternative means that it quickly turns to glucose in the body and upsets blood sugar levels, causing first the symptoms of fatigue associated with low blood sugar and then, if left unchecked, turning eventually into late-onset diabetes? That it also upsets the balance of essential minerals available to the body as well as its acid/alkali balance? And that its lack of fibre means it is one of the main causes of bowel diseases such as diverticulitis?

Do they realise that their daily bread might be making them ill? I once read that ducks on a pond had died when fed with scraps of white bread due to the bleach and chemicals it contained. I cannot vouch for that, but I can well believe it was true!

If, by some means or other, people have become aware of the situation, are they simply depressed or do they realise that there is in fact an answer, that it's *not* too late to improve matters, that something can still be done to ensure the health of our bodies even though we live in an unhealthy environment? The body has amazing recuperative powers if it is given the right fuel for its machinery.

Although changing to a healthy diet is vital, food alone will not supply sufficient nutrients to repair exhausted glands, or ensure the right sort of cholesterol in the arteries once they have started to become blocked and hard, or restore an over-worked immune system. A programme of vitamins and minerals, at therapeutic levels, each in balance with its co-factor nutrients, is needed to undertake this kind of repair work. The damage caused to cells by free radicals can be avoided if the right sort of nutrients, called antioxidants, are available to the body at adequate levels; research indicates that vitamin E will defuse free radical activity in oils and vitamin C will counteract the harmful effects of passive smoking. Specific nutrients will even help to remove traces of mercury from the body of a person who has a mouthful of amalgam fillings!

There is still a chance for our bodies to remain healthy, but we can no longer expect it to happen automatically. We need to know what to do, and then be prepared to make an effort to put our knowledge into practice. The medical profession has discovered a great deal which enables us to live longer lives than our forebears, but we ourselves must be the ones to take responsibility for the *quality* of this life we have been given.

7 A "Rags To Riches" Health Story

I hesitated to include my own story in this book because I was never diagnosed as having M.E. and it therefore might seem inappropriate.

However, looking back over my life I now believe that there were many times when I might well have been given such a diagnosis, but this was twenty, thirty, even forty years ago when the majority of G.P.s did not seem to have heard of M.E. or Chronic Fatigue Syndrome - certainly none that I consulted in all those years.

Even without that diagnosis, I believe that many people who know they have M.E. will identify with much of my story, recognising in their own lives the situations which I describe and thereby finding hope that the outcome for them also might be good.

In addition, I believe there are probably thousands of sick people who, just like me, have not been given a diagnosis and who feel they've been left on the scrap heap and who by some "chance" find themselves reading this book.

These I know will identify with me in the midst of all the uncertainty as to what has gone wrong with their bodies, and I hope that this chapter in particular will show at least a small speck of light at the end of the long, dark tunnel.

As you read, you might be interested to look for the particular pieces of cargo which were weighing down my own good ship *"Immunity"* and causing it to flounder, and see if any of these match up with your own!

Almost sunk without a trace!

I have often said that I could not remember a day in my life when some part of my body did not draw attention to itself.

A "RAGS TO RICHES" HEALTH STORY

This isn't strictly true, for there were many 'sunny' days - playing in fields with childhood friends, Christmas in the cottage where I grew up, teenage fun, falling in love and an Easter wedding, then camping holidays and beach days with the children.

On so many levels, my life was really blessed. The only child of loving parents, the war was going on around and above us but barely touched our lives in the country. I married a loving husband and we had three children who each brought great joy, as did eventually our three children-in-law and four (at the time of writing!) beautiful grandchildren.

Yet much of my life has been a nightmare, for interwoven through it all there was frequent sickness, affecting me not only physically but psychologically, too. There have in fact been very few days in my life when I have been totally free of some kind of illness, pain or anxiety.

Among my earliest memories are ear-ache and thrush as a three-year old. I can remember being sat in a bowl of 'something soothing' with an antiseptic smell, crying because I was so sore. That problem was never away for very long. In addition, I had cold after cold and bilious attack after bilious attack. I was a bright child, doing well at school and enjoying many friendships, and yet the constant pattern of returning to school after illness became a nightmare to me, as time after time I had to rediscover my place in the world of children's relationships. In fact, I remember nothing but kindness and friendship from the village children, but I still dreaded the days when I was well enough to go back to school.

When I passed 'the scholarship' at eleven years old and had to travel daily by train to the Grammar School, I soon developed school phobia. The reason for this, in addition to my constant ill-health, was that I was terrified of the twice-weekly P.E. lessons in case I had to do a somersault, swing over the bar, or hang upside down on apparatus known as ribstalls. I would be physically sick with "nerves" the night before P.E. Eventually there were consultations between my mother and the headmistress, and special arrangements were made for me to be excused from those exercises, but nobody understood my fear - least of all me - or investigated the cause of it. It is only in recent years that I have realised that something was wrong with my balance, causing me to experience dreadful sensations in my head if I was anything but upright and steady.

I was never without good friends, and enjoyed my teenage years. But the heavy colds and bouts of influenza were still frequent and, in my early twenties, I began to suffer from sinusitis. Incredibly, this was not actually diagnosed for years, although I lived for much of the time with a 'spaced out' feeling in my head, which I found hard to describe and no-one could really understand. At one stage the family doctor said I should have a holiday, which I did, but then I developed back pains and an upset tummy, so very little was achieved.

When I married Robin at the age of twenty-three, it was still in the context of constant ill-health which continued to decline, happy though I was. The second year we were married, we lived in London and I was working at the head office of a charity. One day in Spring, I found it increasingly difficult to press the typewriter keys. Trying to ignore it, I went out at lunchtime but felt as though I was having to drag my legs along the pavement. Overcome with panic as to what was happening to me, I was helped back to the office where a taxi was called to take me home and a doctor sent for. Within an hour, I was at a hospital for nervous diseases, being examined by a specialist and a room full of students - but they could find nothing wrong with me!

Robin packed some things and drove me to my parents in the country, where my mother massaged my limbs and slowly, after a few weeks, the strange sensations of numbness and heaviness subsided - only to return in Spring of the following year - and the next, and the next, and the next! Obviously, the whole thing was due to allergy, and I was reacting to some type of pollen. The symptoms were systemic rather than straightforward hayfever or asthma, and therefore difficult for a doctor to diagnose.

The general picture was not improved by dreadful sickness in my three pregnancies, plus the fact that two of the three babies became ill at three weeks old and needed operations for pyloric stenosis. Added to this, just when our third baby became ill, I developed gallstones! The pain I lived through was unbelievable, as I tried to breast-feed a tiny baby who was losing weight because of projectile vomiting. It did not help to be told for six long months by a specialist that the pain was actually caused by post-natal depression!

When baby Hannah was six months old and fully recovered from her operation, I had my gallbladder removed, complete with stones. I went home to start to enjoy my three children. Two months later I was *really* ill! The 'spaced-out' feeling was constant and severe. So were headaches, weak and aching muscles, stomach upsets, palpitations and anxiety. It began quite suddenly. Robin was travelling to Italy on a business trip that day, and I couldn't believe I was feeling so ill just because I was nervous about him going away.

Somehow I struggled on for a year. If I managed to get to a shop at the end of the road, I would have to spend the rest of the day on my bed, too weak to do anything else, my whole body shaking with palpitations. I had to rely on friends and parents to help with the children, taking them to and from school and playgroup. I went away to spend two weeks with an aunt to see if it would help me recover, and at first I felt terrible but by the second week I had definitely started to improve. I returned home feeling hopeful and encouraged but, within a few hours, the symptoms all returned.

One Sunday, I was lying in bed feeling definitely more dead than alive. Robin was trying to look after the children and also find ways of supporting me. I can remember feeling that, in order to stay alive, I needed to concentrate really hard on something - so we played game after game of 'Battleships' on the bed. Robin had sent for the doctor, and eventually an elderly locum arrived.

"How do you feel?" he asked.

"As though I'm dying", was all I could say.

"Sounds like an allergy", said the doctor, immediately.

He pulled up my nightie and, using his thumbnail, drew lines across my tummy. As we watched, the thin scratch marks turned into wide, red weals, which stayed for a good ten minutes.

"Just as I thought", said the doctor. "You can play noughts and crosses on an allergy patient!" And he wrote out a prescription for anti-histamine tablets.

Allergy again!

Once I had got used to the drowsiness they caused, the tablets certainly helped. But what had caused the allergy? No-one seemed particularly bothered or able to find out. It was my mother who came up with an idea some time later.

She suggested that I might be reacting to the new North Sea gas which had been installed in all the houses in our area the previous year. (The talk at the time had been of 'conversion'; "Have you been converted yet?"!)

We laughed at my mother for making such a suggestion, but she insisted that her friend had suffered from really severe asthma ever since her gas supply had been converted. Well, anything was worth a try! It was summer, so the only gas being used in the house was for the cooker. Robin left me with supplies of food and a vacuum flask each morning, so that I could stay out of the kitchen. And by the end of the week I was definitely feeling better! There was no doubt about it, so we quickly arranged to go "all-electric". Not only the gas cooker and heaters were removed, but all the gas pipes under the house. I certainly was very much better - but soon made two more discoveries.

The first was that as soon as I went into other houses or buildings where there was gas, I would be ill for the next four or five days with all the symptoms of 'flu'. It would happen whether I knew there was gas or not. Sometimes I would become ill and we would try to retrace my steps of the previous day - and invariably we would find a gas heater tucked behind a shop counter, or something similar.

The second discovery was that I was now allergic to many other things as well, presumably because I had been exposed to the gas for so long. In particular, the smell of paint would give me a blazing headache and set off all the old symptoms. The worst problem was to find that I had become allergic to local anaesthetics, and the reaction was so severe that for the next seventeen years I had all my dentistry without an anaesthetic, including three crowns in one session!

It took a lot of 'fight' to keep facing up to the constant problems, yet many people made it clear that they thought me a hypochondriac. They had no idea of my constant struggle to find the physical and mental strength which were needed simply to keep myself going.

By 1972, the wear and tear of all I had been through had taken their toll of my body and my nerves. I experienced constant infections - sinusitis, 'flu', tummy bugs, kidney infections, cystitis, thrush, fibrositis, day in and day out. Added to this were the complications caused by the various allergies. Trying to bring up a family of three small children involved a daily battle with my body. I was exhausted, and exhaustion led to an anxiety state for which I was eventually prescribed some tranquillisers.

Allergies were a major problem, particularly in the Spring. Every year for twelve years, from March till July, my arms and legs would feel heavy, weak and numb, and I ached in every possible muscle. It was a time of year I dreaded.

One day in 1972, a friend popped in and dropped a book in my lap.

"See what you think of that!", she said.

The book was LET'S GET WELL[14], by Adelle Davis. I read it with amazement. It talked about all sorts of symptoms and conditions which I knew very well indeed, and it gave advice on how to tackle the problems with diet and vitamins! Until then, I had honestly thought that you ate whatever you most enjoyed, and your body did its own thing! It had never before occurred to me that the two were closely connected!

The tide begins to turn

Adelle Davis's book spoke a lot about which vitamins and minerals could be helpful for specific problems. I found it *extremely* interesting! I decided to try a few of her suggestions. She had written a lot about allergies, for which she recommended large doses of vitamin C and pantothenic acid (vitamin B5) to help counteract the reactions. I tried it and it worked. In fact, it worked better than any of the antihistamine drugs I had ever been prescribed, and without the side-effects of drowsiness. I found that if I took these two supplements at breakfast, in half-an-hour's time I would start to feel very much better. Then towards mid-day the symptoms would start to return, but another dose at lunch-time pushed them away again. Four times daily I needed to take good levels of the two supplements providing vitamin C and pantothenic acid, so the tablets went with me wherever I went, and made all the difference in the world to how I felt! It was truly amazing!

A whole new discovery had opened up to me - that food affects the body! I suddenly realised that food is the fuel which makes our machinery work, just like petrol in a car! The fuel I had put into my body for the past thirty-seven years had probably been about the lowest grade possible. I particularly liked sweet things!

What about coffee, which I drank several times each day? It didn't seem possible that coffee might be affecting my health in adverse ways; after all, it is part of our every-day culture.

I decided to see what would happen if I gave it up for a while. The effect was dramatic and fairly immediate. Cystitis - that wretched complaint which had me sitting in the doctor's waiting room more times than I cared to remember - completely disappeared!

In my discoveries about diet, I found something very interesting indeed! One of the health problems discussed by Adelle Davis was low blood sugar - hypoglycaemia. As I read her case studies, I recognised myself. Very often, by tea-time, I would collapse with what I called 'tea-time tizziness'. Quite suddenly, I would have to sit in a chair, absolutely still, unable even to turn my eyes sideways for fear of 'keeling over' and far too weak to talk.

We had found out what to do about it. As soon as it happened, Robin would prepare a plate of food as quickly as he could and put it on my lap. I would eat it slowly, bite by bite, not moving my head or my eyes, until gradually the food would restore some strength to my body and, after a while, I would be able to cope with putting the children to bed!

From Adelle Davis's description, I was certain that this was hypoglycaemia. She gave some information about how to deal with it, but I needed to know more. It was going to be necessary to think through a radical change in diet, for one thing, and the vitamins and minerals which she recommended required a lot of working out. I needed more help - and it came!

One Sunday morning an unknown lady came and stood next to me in church. After the service, we started to chat. Veronica spoke with an American accent, though I discovered she was English by birth and had married an American and lived there for many years. She had come over from Boston, Massachusetts, for the sad task of putting her elderly mother into a nursing home and selling up the family home and contents. She was in England for a month and very lonely, living in a deserted house with gradually-lessening furniture. I invited her to come to us whenever she liked in the evenings, and we soon became good friends.

It just so happened that Veronica had suffered from hypo-glycaemia but had been completely cured through following a special diet and taking a programme of vitamins and minerals recommended by doctors at an American clinic. She was able to help me with all that I needed to know and, when she returned to America, she sent me several books to help me even further. Among other things, I learned the importance of not eating sugar, and of having a protein snack every two hours. I took more vitamins. And I began to feel very much better! Increasingly, I was coming to understand the way in which food, together with vitamin and mineral supplements, could help my body to function more efficiently.

Slowly, surely, my health was being rebuilt. Yet often there were set-backs and for much of the time I still had sickness or pain. Even though allergies and blood sugar problems were now tremendously improved, it seemed as though there was still one heavy piece of cargo on board my *"Immunity"* ship which was keeping me pretty well submerged! What else did I need to discover?

In 1985 I heard about yeast infection. I was now regularly taking vitamins, which I ordered from a mail order food supplement company. Occasionally, they would enclose fact sheets in the parcel and I would read about various health problems and the way they could be helped therapeutically through diet and food supplements. One of these fact sheets was headed: THE SPORES THAT ATTACK YOU: WHEN YOUR IMMUNE SYSTEM CAN'T PROTECT YOU[15]. The introduction said that a yeast which lives harmlessly in everyone can also cause symptoms as diverse as runny nose, constipation, diarrhoea, bloated stomach, headaches, depression or infections of the vagina, kidneys and bladder. It could also cause many other problems. It was called *Candida albicans*.

Conquering Candida!

My doctor said I could not possibly be suffering from yeast infection because, if I were, it would have cleared up with one week's treatment, which we had already tried for thrush.

However, the fact sheet said something very different, that it was difficult to bring candida under control but that it could be done with dedicated attention to diet (avoiding all yeasts and sugars), the inclusion of several vitamin and mineral supplements, and an anti-fungal drug called Nystatin which might be needed for several months. My doctor would not agree to prescribe the drug for me, so I decided I had to do what I could on my own and try to work out the diet. I stuck to it faithfully, but, although I was convinced that I was on the right lines, the diet on its own made very little difference.

I had a friend called Moira, who also had a great many health problems. We believed that she, too, had 'yeast infection'. She decided to try the diet.

In February 1987, Moira came to me and said,

"Guess what! My GP has become interested in yeast

infection and he wants to meet you!"

This was incredible! I had thought it would be quite impossible to find a doctor who would be interested in hearing what I had discovered, but now here was a doctor wanting to meet me! I arranged to visit him and we spent an interesting hour, pooling our knowledge of *Candida albicans,* and he kindly agreed to take me as a patient. I transferred to his practice and he was happy to prescribe me some Nystatin to try. He also gave me an even stricter diet to follow, which he had recently heard about.

I began to feel unbelievably depressed, to the point of being morbid. My sinuses and ears became extremely painful. I developed appalling pains in my mouth which seemed to come from the nerves in every single tooth and seared right through the roof of my mouth. There were days when I could not lift my face from the pillow because of the intensity of this throbbing pain. Things seemed to be getting worse instead of better.

After a while, I discovered that garlic oil had antifungal properties, and in desperation I tried applying it to my mouth in an attempt to relieve the pain - with very helpful results, initially. I started to 'paint' my mouth with garlic oil each night as I went to bed; fortunately, I have a very long-suffering husband! (I later discovered that garlic was not in fact helping the situation in the long term because of its ability to destroy friendly bacteria as well as yeast! I would now use propolis in this situation.)

This phase passed after a couple of months, and I continued to take Nystatin and keep to the diet. Having come through the bad patch, things seemed to be pretty much as they were before.

At Christmas I went down with some sort of virus infection, and I just couldn't seem to get over it. Week after week, I sat by the fire, aching and with no energy. This had been the pattern so many times before. Some days I would think all day about the breakfast dishes waiting to be washed, but I didn't have the strength to drag myself to the sink. On the rare occasions when I did manage it, I would stand and lean against the draining board, while the muscles in my back and legs just ached and ached and ached. For four months, it took more strength than I could muster to do that one simple task, and this was a situation I could remember happening many times before. I felt so guilty when Robin came home in the evenings and I still hadn't cleared the breakfast things!

By April 1988, I was still no better and I had come to realise that several of my friends, including Moira, were also suffering from the same type of syndrome, to a greater or lesser extent. About that time, I was lent a back copy of HERE'S HEALTH magazine in which there was an appeal by some students at the Institute for Optimum Nutrition for volunteers to take part in a research trial. They were looking into the effectiveness of a natural substance which was *'proving to be dramatically effective against the growing threat of candida albicans infection'*. The magazine was a few weeks out of date, but I quickly wrote off to see if I could volunteer for the trial. Eventually, I received a reply stating that the researchers had found sufficient volunteers, but meanwhile I did some detective work.

I asked every health food shop and every chemist in my area if they had heard of this new substance or of the company (BioCare) which was marketing the product. None of them had, for it turned out to be a very new company, but one chemist kindly spent thirty minutes on the telephone till he tracked them down for me. I wrote to BioCare and asked for information.

They sent me some interesting literature which explained that the product was based on a fatty acid derived from coconuts. It had been known in the 1930s that certain fatty acids had antifungal properties and, in the 1950s, it was found that caprylic acid from coconuts had a fungicidal effect specifically against *Candida albicans*. Caprylic acid products had been researched very thoroughly in America over the previous five years and, at the time of my discovery, they had been available in this country for only a few months. It was recommended that caprylic acid should be taken with other supplements known as probiotics, which would reintroduce some friendly bacteria into the intestines. These I found from a company called Nature's Best.

I sent for both new supplements and carefully read the instructions. The recommendation was that caprylic acid should be taken at top dose straight away (twelve capsules daily) in case strains of yeast were produced which might prove resistant to caprylic acid at lower levels. I started to take them. For nearly three weeks, I noticed nothing - and then something hit me! Another enormous cloud of morbid depression descended upon me, interspersed with bouts of terrible anxiety. My ears became sore and thrush was severe. I ached in every muscle and felt ill all over. I didn't know what was happening, because as yet I had not understood about die-off reaction, so I continued to take all the capsules.

Fortunately, later research showed that high levels of caprylic acid were not in fact necessary to avoid the development of resistant yeasts, so that it was therefore quite safe if taken at low levels. I was very glad to learn this, because it meant that no-one now would ever need to experience the horrendous level of die-off which I had had to endure, caused as it was by tremendously high levels of caprylic acid destroying vast amounts of candida, which in turn released phenomenal numbers of toxins into my body. I vowed that if ever I were to give advice on how to take caprylic acid, it would be to start with low levels and to build it up gradually, as die-off symptoms allowed, and this continues to be a vital part of the advice which I now give, as a qualified Nutritionist, to my candida clients.

After a while, I started to feel better and people noticed a difference in me. They began to ask whether I could help them with their own health problems. I discovered Dr. Crook's candida questionnaire[12] which was a good way of telling whether or not someone's health problems might be due to yeast infection and, if so, to what extent. If they had a high score, I told them about the anti-candida diet I was following and the various supplements they needed.

The real break-through in my health came towards the end of June, about three months after I had started to take caprylic acid and probiotic tablets. Hannah, by then at University in Cardiff, was due home for the long summer holidays. Being the end of the academic year, she needed to bring a lot of her belongings home with her. Somebody had to collect her by car and, as Robin was away on a three-month Christian training course in

Sussex, it had to be me! I had never in my life driven more than a few miles at a time - twenty at the most - because I would so quickly become fatigued and, in any case, my health was so unreliable that it was likely to let me down at any moment! Now I was considering driving over two hundred miles, alone, from Essex to Cardiff, and then back again with Hannah - and I was looking forward to it. Something was very different!

In fact, I stayed two nights in Wales and drove with Hannah for a day's walking in the Brecon Beacons, and the next day we went to a beach on the Gower Peninsular, and on the way home to Essex we went to visit Robin in Horsham. In four days I had driven over nine hundred miles. My health had been fine and I had enjoyed every minute. I even coped with having to call for the AA when my car broke down on the M4 motorway!

Although at that stage I found that I still had recurring thrush and a less-than-perfect immune system, for the most part I now felt well and had more stamina than I could ever remember. There is all the difference in the world between on the one hand being ill and on the other hand being well apart from a few odd symptoms! I felt sure the remaining problems would catch up with the improvements already made before too long.

Nutrition Training

My new-found health was clearly visible and made an impact on many people, including my doctor. I received more and more phone calls from an increasing number of people asking if I could help them, as word seemed to spread like wildfire that I had found an answer to my chronic health problems. Each time I was asked for advice, I was very aware of my dreadfully inadequate knowledge but I also became increasingly conscious of the enormous number of people who were having to put up with chronic ill-health and seeking desperately for answers which the medical profession seemed unable to provide.

One day I came across a notice in HERE'S HEALTH magazine publicising a two-year Diploma Course at the Institute for Optimum Nutrition in London, to provide training for would-be Nutrition Consultants. Was this perhaps what I should do? Would a grandmother be accepted as a student? The course was pretty expensive; could we afford it?

These and other questions kept buzzing round my head, but the idea of training to become a Nutrition Consultant just wouldn't go away. I telephoned the Institute to make some enquiries and was invited to one of their Open Days for an interview. It so happened that I could manage none of the dates they offered, because of family holidays or other prior engagements, and I expressed disappointment. However, after a few more questions, I was offered an interview by telephone, which seemed second-best but at least would enable me to follow through with the possibility of training.

The interview went well and I was offered a place for the Autumn term. What *had* I done? How much study would I have to do, and to what standard? I had left school at seventeen with some good O-levels and then had taken a secretarial and languages course at the City of London College, where I achieved some R.S.A. certificates. That had been the extent of my academic career, and it had ended thirty-five years ago! With this humble level of educational achievement, which was below the normal requirements for the I.O.N. course, I had been given to understand that the reason I had been accepted was because of my obvious knowledge and enthusiasm for the subject and the fact that I was already involved in giving basic nutritional advice to many people who were requesting it. The interviewer obviously felt that I was the right sort of material to become a Nutrition Consultant!

One of the requirements of the Institute was that students without a scientific background should first of all enrol for a five-week science foundation course to study the basics of biochemistry. I didn't even have a science subject among my O-levels, so I certainly needed to do this basic study. I went to London for the first weekend of the course, and came home with my mind completely boggled! I was having to learn a whole new scientific language, and to wrap my mind around some completely new and bewildering concepts. Was I going to be struggling like this through two long years? I was grateful that my husband had a degree in Natural Sciences from Cambridge, and that for the past thirteen years he had been teaching science to A-level students.

I had to ask him some pretty basic questions, and he patiently helped me to understand. Towards the end of the five weeks, we spent the school half-term in our caravan in Wales, and devoted part of every day to going through my heavy textbooks. Robin says that to start with we were talking first-year secondary school science, but by the end of five weeks we were at first-year university level! My brain had received a kick-start and was getting nicely into gear.

I had enrolled at I.O.N. as a 'satellite' student, which meant that the regular lectures were sent to me on tapes. I studied at home and submitted my work by post, but I also had to attend the Institute for several weekends in the year for workshops or seminars with my group tutor, Patrick Holford.

Having completed the science foundation course, I looked at the syllabus of work ahead and felt utterly overwhelmed. It covered all the major body systems and the part played by specific nutrients in the efficient functioning of each system. In addition, there would be lectures on such things as helping the body to deal with the effects of pollution, the politics of the food industry, when to refer clients to their doctor, etc., etc. It also covered workshops on giving public presentations and preparing press releases and many other aspects of working as a Nutrition Consultant. We would of course be learning how to calculate nutritional requirements from an analysis of symptoms in a client's questionnaire, and how to formulate an appropriate tailor-made supplement programme. It was all going to be extremely interesting, but there was so much of it! At the end of each of the two years there would be an examination, the final one covering the whole two years' work, and in the second year it would be necessary to submit case studies of thirty-eight clients, some with three-month and six-month follow-ups. Most worrying of all, in the second year we would have to plan, carry out and write up a research project!

The reading list was heavy, literally! We bought some bookshelves and a desk from a second-hand shop and these were put into our smallest bedroom, which was fast becoming a cross between a study and an office because, besides studying, I was also getting busier in another direction! People were growing well through following my elementary nutritional advice, even though as yet I knew so little, but word of mouth was spreading and we were beginning to get telephone calls from people where we couldn't even trace the contact! The small bedroom needed a filing cabinet and a card index system on the desk.

At one stage our local paper carried a disparaging article about M.E. entitled, YUPPIE FLU, and I was incensed enough to write a letter explaining what I had so far discovered. As a result, I was interviewed and an article was printed - which triggered so much interest that two weeks later a second article was run and this time, without my knowledge, it gave my telephone number.

In the next two days I received seventy-two phonecalls from people desperate for help. I told them as much as I could, and agreed to obtain antifungal supplements for them if they asked me to. The telephone never stopped ringing, and we had to leave it off the hook at mealtimes in order to have some peace, so the next things needed were an answerphone and a second telephone line to make it possible for our family to get through to us!

The growing numbers of consultations and letters to distant people were taking up a lot of time, so that my studying frequently had to be done very late at night, and yet my stamina didn't give out. I still had a few minor symptoms, but basically I was *well!* I had never before experienced such ongoing good-health, yet just a few months earlier it had seemed quite impossible that I would ever again have energy to wash the dishes!

Homework marks began to come in, and they were encouraging. Perhaps I could do it, after all! I found I enjoyed studying. For my research project, I chose to set up a trial on a nutritional approach for eating disorders. I had already seen how anorexia and bulimia could shatter the lives both of sufferers and their families, but I had also seen how nutrition, in particular the use of broad-spectrum amino acid supplements, had made a tremendous difference in the few cases where I had been asked for advice. I was glad to have an opportunity to test my findings on a wider scale, and to strengthen my growing conviction that most eating disorder situations had a *physical* cause at their root, and not just a psychological cause as was generally accepted.

I co-opted help from the local press to find volunteers, and eventually had some very encouraging results. One lady, who had suffered with bulimia for thirty years and also with severe multiple joint pain, was completely free of both conditions after just ten weeks' nutritional guidance!

During those two years of study and increasing requests for help, I coped with several family responsibilities, as well. Grand-daughter Grace was born, and I spent ten days helping out in Emma's household. My mother was twice in hospital, severely ill with pancreatitis, and I managed to visit her daily and also look after her flat. Hannah needed someone to type her project report for her degree in Ophthalmic Optics so I did it for her in the Easter break. Somehow everything got done, and my strength held out.

The two years flew by, culminating in October 1990 with my graduation. Out of forty-six students completing the course, I had come first - a clear sign that hard work and enthusiasm pay off! Meanwhile, the consultancy work continued to snowball, and we decided it was time to "go for it". Robin handed in his notice at school and joined me to take over administration of the practice. My friend Moira had been helping in the office and was a tremendous support throughout. Having a four-bedroomed house and our children all flown from the nest, we were able to use one bedroom as a consulting room and one as an office. We had to think of systems to cope with the workload, and our son Toby, now living with his family near Leeds, designed some helpful programmes for us on a small computer. Before long a team of assistants began to grow, until at the time of writing there are eight of us needed to cope with the workload, including typists, receptionists and people to despatch orders for supplements. We also aim to take on more professional help from other qualified Nutritionists.

Three years after qualifying, I undertook an additional year of study because the basic ION course had been extended to three years and I wanted to upgrade my qualification accordingly. For my required dissertation, I wrote about the controversy surrounding candidiasis and a nutritional approach to its management. By the time I had looked at available research papers and medical text books, and was questioned on the contents of my dissertation for the final Viva examination, I began to feel as though I knew about candida inside-out!

I was invited to lecture at the Institute on what had become my two "pet subjects" of Candidiasis and M.E.; later, I went on to lecture in Practice Management and Client/Consultant Relationships. What a long way I had come in a short space of time! For two years I also tutored third year students, but eventually I found that this was just a little too much to fit in with my very demanding workload, so I sadly resigned as tutor - partly, I must admit, as a minor concession to the fact that I had reached the age of sixty!

In 1990, Gill Jacobs (now on the Council of Management of *Action for M.E. and Chronic Fatigue*) contacted me and asked if she could include my story in a book she was writing, to be entitled, CANDIDA ALBICANS; YEAST AND YOUR HEALTH.[16] This led to a large number of enquiries, many from people who said, *"Your story has such a happy ending!"*. In 1994, Gill updated her book under a new title, CANDIDA ALBICANS: A USER'S GUIDE TO TREATMENT AND RECOVERY,[17] but she kept my story in it and it still brings in a large number of enquiries.

Another book, THE PRACTICAL GUIDE TO CANDIDA,[18] by Jane McWhirter, published in 1995, makes gracious comments about both my work and the BEAT CANDIDA COOKBOOK[1], leading to even more interest. Leon Chaitow's book, CANDIDA ALBICANS: COULD YEAST BE YOUR PROBLEM?,[19] published in 1985, was the first book on the British scene and remains a classic. It is good that the role of candida in chronic health problems is being placed increasingly on the map by writers such as Leon, Gill and Jane who each has an excellent understanding of the problem although differing in some details of their advice from my own.

In 1991, I wrote and published the BEAT CANDIDA COOKBOOK[1] initially just to help my clients but it soon became popular with other sufferers and practitioners also. I quickly managed to develop a technique for undertaking consultations by post, which means that I am able to advise clients around the country and even overseas, and my typists are kept busy preparing reports and letters which explain my findings and recommendations based on analysis of their completed questionnaires.

I receive encouraging feedback not only from clients but also occasionally from their doctors and specialists. I have been involved with various conditions, including heart disease and schizophrenia, where there has been approving comment from the hospital Consultant involved. My favourite remark was made by a doctor in Yorkshire who, on seeing the report I had sent to his patient said, *"This lassie knows what she's on about!"*

Nutritionists do not claim to have a cure for any illness, but they do claim to be able to help each person achieve a status of optimum nutrition where many health problems simply cannot exist. It is obvious that both the body and the mind will work more efficiently if they are optimally nourished - which means supplying necessary levels of each nutrient to repair damaged cells and correct biochemical imbalances.

More about Candida

When I first learned about *Candida albicans,* it was like finding a missing piece of jigsaw puzzle. It explained so many things which had been happening in my body.

For one thing, I discovered that this yeast seems to love to inhabit old injury sites such as knees or back. At the age of eighteen, I had fallen down some concrete steps onto a station platform, causing excruciating pain and severe bruising. After five years of suffering from repeated episodes of "slipped disc", I was eventually shown by an osteopath that one of my vertebrae had been knocked sideways. (Several hospital specialists had failed to spot this on the X-rays.) Although osteopathic treatment and exercise helped me to recover from the initial injury, it left me with an extremely weak and painful spine for many years. Since candida has been under control in my body, I have virtually forgotten the problems with my back which recurred with depressing regularity for more than thirty years!

I came to understand why I had to abandon any attempts to make bread or wine, even though at one time we bought ourselves jars and corks and all the paraphernalia of a wine-making kit! The incredibly severe headaches which flattened me on each occasion meant it was quite impossible to continue with our wine-making dream. Now I knew it was because the overgrowth of yeast in my body had made my immune system hypersensitive to the smell of yeast in my environment.

And I discovered that there were, in fact, other people like me who had become allergic to local anaesthetics, in spite of the fact that one dental specialist told me that this was simply not possible and that quite obviously I was the type of woman who fainted when I saw the needle! (I couldn't help wondering how *he* would cope if he had to have three teeth drilled and crowns fitted all in one session without the luxury of a local anaesthetic, as I once did!)

Whilst on the subject of teeth, at one stage my dentist advised me to have some old crowns removed and replaced. They had moved very slightly over the years, leaving a small gap below the gum line. I felt that candida might be hiding inside these crowns, because if ever I had a flare-up of old symptoms, it always started in that area of my mouth. As the old crowns were removed, I could *smell* the infection inside them. Whether this was fungal or bacterial, I don't know, but either way it meant that my immune system had fewer battles on its hands once my nice new teeth were firmly in place!

Other people also reported severe reactions to medicines and drugs prescribed by the doctor, just as I had so often experienced. For me, antibiotics created a horrendous sense of panic, and I remember nights when I walked round and round the bedroom in an attempt to keep my sanity, yet the panic subsided as soon as the effects of the antibiotic wore off. On one occasion, the doctor prescribed some pills for a tummy upset. In a very short space of time I felt as though the room had gone dark. I could hardly see and I could barely move. I crawled on all fours to the telephone and managed to gasp out to my doctor what was happening to me. He seemed not at all perturbed and told me to eat some bread and marmite, for what reason I was never clear! After some hours, the effects began to go and it was as though a light had been switched on in the room and I could see again. I was left feeling weak and grey, and vowed never to touch that particular drug again!

When I first learned about candida and became convinced that this was the basic cause of all my problems, it came as a great relief. For years I had felt that I was disintegrating in all directions; now I knew there was just one major problem for which I needed to find the answer.

I realised, too, that although the vitamins I had been taking for several years had played a significant part in my recovery, it would have been much more effective had I known exactly what to take and how much of it! I knew that this boosting of the immune system had to be a vital part of any strategy which attempted to overcome candida.

So, both from my experience and from the training I had received, I found I had put together a four-point plan to recommend to other candida sufferers. Increasingly, as I gave this advice, I saw an astonishing number of people becoming well. The first time I tried to help someone who had been medically diagnosed as having M.E., I realised that candida was largely responsible for his illness, if not totally. This was a man in his early forties who had been unable to work for over two years and could just about manage to walk from his car with the aid of a stick. After five months on a nutritional anti-candida regime, he was able to return to work!

He was the first of many, but I found that for some it takes a considerably longer time. These folk require even greater measures of patience, perseverance and determination. I have known a very few people who became well in just three months; others have taken over a year, especially if they have been housebound or even bed-bound for a long time beforehand. The experience of most people with candidiasis falls somewhere in between, taking them perhaps six to nine months or even up to a year to feel completely well. It is impossible to say in advance how long it will take, because everyone is so completely different. People who have never taken the Pill or used steroids and who do not smoke will usually recover more quickly than those whose history is full of immune-suppressing medication or alcohol or drugs and those who are determined to keep on smoking!

Yeast infection is a wretched complaint from beginning to end, for even the process of getting rid of it is no joy-ride. How good to know that we *can* break free of its hold on our lives!

Sailing Free!

The understanding I have gathered regarding a nutritional approach to overcoming health problems came about first of all as the result of my own improvements in health, followed by three years of training in Optimum Nutrition and then increasing experience as I have seen an enormous number of people respond to nutritional advice. For me, it has been like living an adventure story which became more and more exciting as I turned the pages! How did it all come about? There is just one answer; through faith.

Alongside my story of physical discoveries, there also ran an exciting thread of growing awareness in my spiritual life. Although I had been a Christian for many years, I still had a great deal to learn about God's love and power and his desire to bless me with health and in other ways, but that's another story which would fill another book!

However, I am ending this particular small volume by

discussing a nutritional approach from a Christian viewpoint. The first seven chapters are complete in themselves, and I do not wish to persuade you to read the final chapter unless you have a specific interest in considering my thoughts on another aspect of healing and wholeness.

If you end your reading here, I hope you have been inspired by my own "rags to riches" story (in terms of health!) and that you now feel it might conceivably be possible to find some light at the end of your own particular tunnel.

Whether or not my years of illness could or should have been diagnosed and labelled as M.E., I am certain that many who read this book will have identified with at least some of the suffering and symptoms which I experienced, and will have recognised in themselves the pieces of cargo which were placing a load on my particular *"Immunity"* - allergy, pollution, low blood sugar, stress, nutritional deficiencies and candida, at the very least!

With such pieces of cargo - and possibly others - identified in your own life and then off-loaded, I pray that you, too, will be able to "sail free", as I have done!

8 Nutrition: In Line With God

Life in a fallen world

None of the problems associated with pollution, pesticides and depleted diet existed when God first created man and put him on planet Earth, neither did they exist when Jesus lived in Galilee. Most of them didn't even exist as recently as the last century!

With increasing scientific knowledge and skill, mankind has managed to mess up his environment and his food. As a result, malnutrition is not confined to Third World countries, as we tend to suppose, and the health of the Western world is spiralling downwards. A great many health problems are now accepted as being a normal part of life but simply do not occur when the body is optimally nourished.

For example, I have found that the majority of women expect to suffer the monthly miseries of P.M.T., yet I have also found many times over that when diets are improved and nutritional deficiencies and imbalances corrected, the same women who regularly dissolved into tears or screamed at their husbands and children for part of every month (and felt guilty the rest of the time!) now do not even notice their period starting and are able to remain the affectionate wives and mothers they really are. The accepted monthly trauma does not *need* to happen, and *will* not happen if women learn to take care of their hormonal machinery by returning as closely as possible to the original eating plan and doing everything possible to offset the effects on their bodies of environmental pollution.

They need to realise that it's the coffee they drink to keep them going (or the chocolate bars grabbed between meals, or the left-over cake finished up as they clear the table!), together with a general lack of good nutritious food which is actually causing them to feel and behave the way they do.

Getting to grips

We need to get to grips with the situation, and, as a Christian myself, I believe that Christians should take a lead in this! It has been quite clear in my own life that God wanted me to understand the importance of being a proper "steward" of my body, learning to treat it with the respect it deserves. Whatever I might think of it when I look in the mirror, it is in fact a quite amazing piece of handiwork! According to the Bible, it is also a temple of the Holy Spirit. (see 1 Corinthians 3:16)

My experience of sickness into health enabled my body, as well as my soul and my spirit, to come into line with the truth of God's word in the Bible when it says, *"Through his wounds you have been healed"*. (1 Peter 2:24). God's healing is given by grace (in other words, he freely gives us what we don't deserve and haven't had to earn), but that doesn't excuse us from living a life of faith and obedience.

When I reflect on my story and consider how many Christians are now being led to contact me for nutritional advice, I cannot help but see God's hand in it.

It is also no accident that you are reading this book - at least, if you believe that God guides our lives, as I do. So what do you think is the purpose behind it?

Perhaps God wants to help you take hold of healing for yourself or for someone near to you through a nutritional approach like the one outlined in earlier chapters. I believe - and I hope you do, too - that God can heal in an instant if he chooses, yet for some reason there are times when he apparently decides to heal us through getting us to change our diet and take some vitamins!

Why should this be? Is it because he knows we need more self-discipline? That was definitely a need in my life, and keeping to a strict diet certainly increases self-control! What better motivation could you have than to know that through it you will not only become healthy but that you are also pleasing God?

Perhaps there is a challenge for you; do you really *want* to be well? This might seem a ridiculous question, but Jesus once asked it of a man who had been ill for thirty-eight years, so he must have known that sometimes it needs to be asked. (John 5:6). When Jesus heard his answer, that man was healed *"at once"*, the Bible says!

If Jesus asked you the same question, you might reply, "Lord, you *know* I want to be well, but I couldn't possibly give up eating bread, or drinking tea, or eating chocolate" ... or whatever else it might take to restore you to health.

He asks again, *"Do you want to be well?"*

Perhaps he wants you to trust him more for your needs? Food supplements - and, I'm afraid, professional advice - cost money. If you believe that God is leading you to nutritional help for your healing, should you really be saying, "Oh, but I couldn't afford it!"? I have seen many times how he undertakes the financial cost for someone who looks to him for provision, confirming in the process that this is the way he has chosen for their healing. (Here I will say that there was a time when everything I recommended in a supplement programme could be obtained on an NHS prescription if a doctor was willing to co-operate, but Government cuts have led to very few items now being prescribable. Although this is tragic, God will have a way for you to afford all that he wants you to have. He never asks us to do something without also giving us the resources to do it!)

Possibly God simply wants you to learn about the importance of good nutrition, so that your future life can be lived in health and not in constant need of healing? Is he concerned that, if you are a wife and mother, you should think more responsibly about the food you feed to your family, so that in years to come your husband will not keel over with a sudden heart attack, your teenage daughter will not succumb to anorexia and your elderly mother fall prey to brittle bones or senile dementia? So much can be done to avoid each of these tragic situations. And if you yourself are approaching the menopause, do you really think God intended that this stage of life should need the help of artificial hormones?

Can we, before God, put our heads in the sand and do nothing about improving our own health and that of our families, simply because we don't want to give up eating the foods we like or deprive our families of the things they have grown to enjoy?

Perhaps you have thought it makes no difference whether you eat brown bread or white. Possibly, even, you have laughed at those who will eat only brown! But wouldn't you rather eat the sort of wholesome food that Jesus ate? White bread is of no value to our bodies; in fact it is positively harmful! Food is meant to do us good, not fill us with rubbish and man-made chemicals and additives.

God said, '*See, I give you all the seed-bearing plants that are upon the whole earth, and all the trees with seed-bearing fruit; this shall be your food.*' (Genesis 1:29)

He also said, '*Every living and crawling thing shall provide food for you, no less than the foliage of plants.*' (Genesis 9:3)

He provided us with good things to eat, and nowhere did he say, 'Go and mix up some chemicals to add to it, and refine the flour to remove its goodness'!

In line with God's wishes

I believe that Christians need to realise how much we have abused our bodies so that we can ask forgiveness and then learn anew how to live in ways which are pleasing to God. We will then be co-operating with him for the physical part of that fullness of life which Jesus has promised us (John 10:10), and our bodies will be submitted to him in the same way as our spirits and our minds.

The apostle John, writing to his friend Gaius, said, '*Dear friend, I am praying that all is well with you and that your body is as healthy as I know your soul is*'. (3 John 1:2, Living Bible)

John would never have prayed something which was not in line with God's wishes; our Father *wants* us to be healthy!

Love God; honour and obey him in every way you can. Love your neighbour; let him see you radiating joy and peace and well-being, physical and mental as well as spiritual, then tell him how he can be the same at every level! Love yourself and your family; show it by changing your shopping habits, start to read labels, learn all you can about healthy food and re-think your lifestyle to include relaxation and exercise. Ask God to help you with these every-day decisions. Invite him into your radical re-think. I am certain he will show you what he wants you to do! And when he makes it clear, show him your love and gratitude by doing what he asks.

Read this promise and claim it for yourself, as I did:

'The Lord will keep all sickness far from you; he will not afflict you with those evil plagues of Egypt which you have known.' (Deuteronomy 7:15, Jerusalem Bible)

But there is a condition for this promise which, if you read the preceding verses, you will find is wrapped up in just one word: obedience.

People sometimes argue that we all have to die some time, so there seems little point in denying ourselves the foods we enjoy just in case they happen to make us ill. I hope you agree with me that this attitude is hardly worth the paper it is printed on! Of course we shall die; nothing is more certain! But death does not have to come through sickness and pain. It should happen simply because our Father has called us home. Many of us have known elderly relatives who have somehow recognised their time to go, peacefully accepted it, and then just fallen asleep - to wake in a better place! And that's how I believe it is meant to be.

Meanwhile, we are all meant to *live!*

Attitudes and choices

I believe that God is challenging all Christians about their attitudes to food. At the very least, he is wanting to sharpen up our self-control. Without realising it, we eat for our own pleasure, for self-gratification, even though we might have given every other area of our lives to God for *his* pleasure. Fasting is encouraged in the Bible, but exercising control over the amount and type of food we eat can actually be harder than a total fast!

In addition, I believe God wants us to use our renewed minds (Romans 12:2) to make proper choices so that our bodies also might be renewed. The trouble is that this generation, through increased advertising and packaging pressure from the food industry, has come to regard as 'normal' whichever foods have the longest shelf-life, the greatest visual appeal, or the most addictive contents. There is nothing normal about such foods, except in the sense that they are eaten by the greatest number of people for the greater part of the time!

So what *should* we eat?

You really don't need me to tell you that the foods which are best for you are those which are completely natural, as God intended - fresh fruit and vegetables, whole grains made into delicious bread and pastry, many kinds of beans and pulses, nuts and seeds, eggs, low fat dairy produce - and, unless you are a vegetarian, organic lean meat (which has not been adulterated with hormones, antibiotics and colouring), free-range poultry and any type of fish.

Why should those who eat food out of packets and drink out of cans be scornful of those who choose to eat *proper* food, knowing that this is the fuel which was specially designed for our bodies? As television advertising makes an increasing impact, isn't it time that Christians took a stand and refused to have their thinking and their spending moulded by the world? Paul says, '*Let your behaviour change, modelled by your new mind. This is the only way to discover the will of God and know what is good, what it is that God wants, what is the perfect thing to do*'. (Romans 12:2 Jerusalem Bible)

Very often people say, "*I'm a great believer in having a little of what you fancy! I can't cope with the idea of watching what I eat. Anyway, I'm never ill, so it must work!*"

They somehow manage to say it with a fair degree of pride, as though they themselves are responsible for this happy state of affairs! They should instead praise God that he is keeping them healthy and that, as yet, he has not asked them to exercise more self-discipline. In any case, the situation will probably not continue all their lives because, after all, machinery is machinery and will not run indefinitely on low-grade fuel. It will either slow down and need lots of servicing, or else it will come to a sudden grinding halt! Unexpected heart attacks or strokes can happen largely because the diet has been deficient in magnesium, which is needed to enable muscles to relax after contracting. If muscles around the heart or an artery go into spasm, and there is not enough magnesium available to relax them, the consequences will be dire.

Magnesium is found in most dark green leafy vegetables (not spinach), dried fruit, some fresh fruit, nuts, seeds, whole grains - in other words, many of the foods which go to make a healthy diet. However, if too much calcium is supplied (from many of the same sources but also from milk products), the balance is tipped and muscles will more easily contract than relax. Too much cheese and other milky products alongside too few green vegetables, nuts and seeds could well lead to a scenario of muscle spasm blocking oxygen supply to the heart or brain. Some diet-related diseases give gradual warnings; with others there is no second chance.

Healing or Health?

Another opinion frequently expressed is that God would prefer to heal through prayer than through alternative therapies. My view is that God is God and will no doubt heal as he chooses! In any case, good nutrition should not be regarded as an alternative therapy. We are not talking about medicine, either orthodox or alternative, although the biochemical understanding of nutrition is in line with 'straight' Western medicine. We are talking about *food*. God might ask us to fast occasionally, but most of the time he expects us to eat! So although I agree that he is more than willing to heal through prayer or Christian ministry, I also believe that he would rather we learned how to be healthy.

It was a wonderful idea on God's part to give us delicious food as fuel rather than a substance like petrol! Vitamin and mineral supplements are just a way of taking food in concentrated form when our bodies need some extra help. It would be great if they were not necessary, but unfortunately in these days of heavy pollution (when even organically grown vegetables contain harmful chemicals from the soil, carried there by contaminated rain) and adulterated food, our bodies need every bit of help they can get to cope with the situation and stay strong.

In some ways it did more harm than good when scientists identified the specific vitamins and minerals present in food, because many people then thought (and still do!) that they could continue with their bad diet and make up for it by taking a few pills. *Nothing* can make up for a poor diet if we want to keep or regain our health.

For more than forty years I ate a diet high in sugar, fat, stimulants and refined grains, with devastating consequences. Within a comparatively short time of realising what I had been doing to myself and radically rethinking my eating habits, I came into a life so 'abundant' that sometimes I say, "Oh, Lord, does it have to be *this* full?" Yet I rejoice in my new-found stamina, which has given me better health at sixty years old than I had at twenty or even ten!

Jesus once healed a blind man who later said, when questioned, *"I only know that I was blind and now I can see"*. (John 9:25). I can identify with that!

When I discovered that I was suffering from yeast infection, I received the laying-on of hands several times from faith-filled Christians who prayed that I might be healed of this specific illness. Each time I received an assurance that the healing *would* come, but that it would be in God's time and so I had to trust him. I believe utterly that he could have healed me on the spot on any of those occasions, but he chose to do it a longer way through teaching me about the importance of good nutrition.

God is a God of love and mercy and has supernatural ability to heal, but I believe that he also asks us to take responsibility for those areas of our lives which he has entrusted to us, which includes our physical bodies. For why should he heal a man of lung cancer who refuses to give up smoking? And why should he heal a woman of obesity and heart disease if her daily food consists of chips, pizza or burgers, with ice-cream and doughnuts to follow and coffee or cola to wash it all down?!

Outsmarting the enemy!

By hearing what God is saying in these days of increasing pollution and undermined bodily defences, we can give the enemy less opportunity to invade our bodies with sickness and disease. We know that he will do whatever he can to make us ineffective as Christian witnesses and, although peace and patience from God might be seen in one who is suffering, the sickness itself does nothing at all for God's honour.

When I realised that our enemy the devil wages warfare against us, I was glad to discover the armour which God provides for our protection. (Ephesians 6:10-16) By beginning to co-operate with God in taking care of my body, I made a stand against the enemy's tactics in the physical realm. That second helping of pudding or 'just one more' chocolate biscuit are probably the most common temptations which most of us experience in our everyday lives. It is no coincidence that man's very first sin was to eat a tempting piece of forbidden fruit! The pleasure we derive from food plays an enormous part in our lives, and the devil knows what he is doing. For one thing, he knows it is much harder for us to fight once he has already weakened our bodies, and it even becomes a battle to pray when we are in the grips of pain or sickness.

Let us determine to thwart the enemy's attempts to ruin our lives and make us ineffective as Christians. Illness is no witness to God's love and power. If that's all you get for being a Christian, who wants to know?

But Jesus says, *"Do you want to be well?"*

Do you want to be well?

Do you?

If so, and you put your faith in Jesus and do whatever he asks you to do, then the Bible promises that he will heal you. Whether your healing comes quickly as a supernatural answer to prayer, or whether it comes slowly as you obey him and persevere, the outcome is equally sure and the glory will go to God!

I have no desire to build false hopes in you. *I* do not make these promises. They are spoken by Jesus Christ himself.

"Whatever you ask in my name, believe that you have received it, and it will be yours." (Mark 11:24)

Why don't you try believing him?

'In all their affliction he was afflicted, and he personally saved them. In his love and pity he redeemed them and lifted them up and carried them through all the years.' Isaiah 63: 9 (Living Bible)

M.E.: SAILING FREE

REFERENCES & RECOMMENDED READING

Introduction

1. White, Erica, "Beat Candida Cookbook", Whites' Food Supplement Supplies, Leigh-on-Sea, Essex, 1993.

Chapter One

2. Loria, R.M., "Coxsachieviruses: A General Update", Plenum, 1988, quoted by D. Jones in What Doctors Don't Tell You, 6:9, December 1995.

3. Jones, Doris, "How vaccines can cause M.E." in What Doctors Don't Tell You, 6:9, December 1995.

Chapter Two

4. Colby, Jane, "M.E.: A polio by another name", in What Doctors Don't Tell You, 6:9, December 1995.

5. Chaitow, Leon, "Post Viral Fatigue Syndrome", Dent, London, 1989.

6. Pauling, Linus, The Last Interview, in Optimum Nutrition, 7:2, Winter 1994.

7. Davies, Stephen and Stewart, Alan, "Nutritional Medicine", Pan Books, London, 1987.

8. Langer, S.E. and Scheer, J.F., "Solved - The Riddle of Illness", Keats Publishing, New Canaan, Connecticut, 1984.

9. Chaitow, Leon, "Beat Fatigue Workbook", Thorsons, 1988.

10. Odds, F.C., "Candida and Candidosis", Bailliere Tindall, London, 1988.

11. White, Erica, "Candidiasis", Lamberts Healthcare Ltd., Tunbridge Wells, 1993.

12. Crook, William G., "The Yeast Connection: A Medical Breakthrough", 2nd ed., Professional Books, Jackson, Tennessee, 1984.

Chapter Three

13. Holford, Patrick, "Optimum Nutrition", ION Press, London, 1992.

Chapter Seven

14. Davis, Adelle, "Let's Get Well", Unwin Paperbacks, London, 1985.

15. Bredell, Frank, "The Spores that Attack You: When Your Immune System Can't Protect You", Felmore Limited Health Publications, Tunbridge Wells. (undated)

16. Jacobs, Gill, "Candida albicans: Yeast and Your Health", Macdonald Optima, London, 1990.

17. Jacobs, Gill, "Candida albicans: a user's guide to treatment and recovery", Optima, London, 1994.

18. McWhirter, Jane, "The Practical Guide to Candida", All Hallows House Foundation, 1995.

19. Chaitow, Leon, "Candida albicans: Could Yeast be Your Problem?", Thorsons, 1985.

Chapter Eight

All scripture references are taken from "The Holy Bible, New International Version", Hodder and Stoughton, unless otherwise stated.

Other versions referred to are:
"The Jerusalem Bible", Darton, Longman and Todd, and
"The Living Bible", Kingsway Publications.

Recommended Reading:
Urquhart, Colin, "Receive Your Healing", Hodder and Stoughton, 1986.

ANTI-CANDIDA DIET

☹ FOODS TO AVOID:

☹ **SUGAR** in all its forms, and food containing sugar. This includes brown or white sugar, demarara, molasses, syrup, honey, malt, chocolate and all other forms of confectionery, icing, marzipan, ice-cream, desserts and puddings, cakes and biscuits, soft drinks including squash and all canned drinks, tinned fruit in syrup, etc. Check all tins and packets for hidden sugar - even some frozen and tinned vegetables! Types of sugar include fructose, lactose, maltose, sucrose and dextrose.

☹ **YEAST** - all food containing it or derived from it. This includes bread, food coated in breadcrumbs, Marmite, Vecon, Bovril, Bisto, Oxo, etc., citric acid, monosodium glutamate, vitamin tablets unless the label specifically states 'yeast-free', citric acid, pizza bases and most makes of pitta bread. Beware of commercial wrapped bread which claims to have no added yeast if it has been made with sourdough or sprouted grains because these products have been fermented and contain their own naturally-produced yeasts.

☹ **REFINED GRAINS** - white flour, granary flour (which is white flour with malt and added whole grains), white rice, white pasta, cornflour, custard powder, cornflakes and cereals unless 'whole grain' or 'wholemeal' is stated.

☹ **MALTED PRODUCTS** - some cereals (e.g. Weetabix), brown Ryvita, granary bread, malted drinks like Ovaltine, Horlicks and Caro.

☹ **ANYTHING FERMENTED** - alcoholic drinks, ginger beer, vinegar and foods containing vinegar (ketchups, pickles, salad cream, baked beans), soya sauce and sourdough bread.

☹ **COW'S MILK** and most milk products, including cream and most cheeses. (See following note about yoghurt and cottage cheese.)

☹ **FRESH FRUIT,** raw, stewed, jam or juice. Fruit juice is pure fructose and often very high in mould! (Exception: freshly-squeezed lemon juice is allowed in salad dressing, sauces, etc., and slices of scrubbed lemon may be added to mineral water.)

☹ **DRIED FRUIT,** including prunes and the fruit in muesli.

☹ **NUTS** - unless freshly cracked - especially peanuts and peanut butter, which contain a lot of mould.

☹ **SMOKED OR CURED** fish and meat, including ham, bacon and smoked salmon, smoked mackerel.

☹ **MUSHROOMS,** which are a fungus. (So are truffles!)

☹ **TEA AND COFFEE** - even decaffeinated, because they still contain other drugs. Also avoid HOT CHOCOLATE.

☹ **COLA DRINKS AND LUCOZADE;** they both contain caffeine, as do BEECHAM'S POWDERS AND SOME PAINKILLERS (e.g. Anadin, Phensic, Panadol Extra).

☹ **ARTIFICIAL SWEETENERS,** which have been found to feed candida just as effectively as sugar, and in any case keep your sweet tooth alive!

☹ **PRESERVATIVES,** which are frequently derived from yeasts and in any case introduce chemicals to the body. (N.B. Sausages, even without preservatives, are high in animal fat and refined cereal.)

NOTE: Some medications encourage the growth of yeast - antibiotics, steroids, the contraceptive pill and hormone replacement therapy, in particular.

☺ FOODS TO ENJOY:

☺ **YEAST-FREE SODA BREAD** made with wholewheat flour or other grains (see recipes). Some bakers will make a batch for your freezer.

☺ **RICE CAKES** (may be lightly toasted), OAT CAKES (malt-free), ORIGINAL or SESAME RYVITA (not brown, it's malted), WHOLEWHEAT CRISPBREADS (read labels carefully).

☺ **PASTRY** made with wholemeal flour, oatmeal and sunflower or olive oil, in proportions of 3:2:2. Make very moist with plenty of water and dust well with flour before rolling

☺ **SOYA MILK** or **RICE DREAM** as milk alternatives. (Different makes of soya milk have very different flavours.)

☺ **BUTTER** in small amounts for spreading or cooking; otherwise for cooking use extra virgin olive oil.

☺ **UNHYDROGENATED MARGARINE:** Granose have a range of different ones, otherwise new-style Flora is pretty good.

☺ **COLD-PRESSED OILS:** sunflower, safflower, linseed, for salad dressings mixed with lemon juice, and with an egg for mayonnaise.

☺ **NATURAL YOGHURT** Low-fat, unflavoured: try it for dessert or breakfast with lecithin granules or a cereal like whole puffed rice. Spread it on top of wholewheat lasagne dishes before baking, or flavour with mint as a dip.

☺ **COTTAGE CHEESE,** as a spread or a filler for your jacket potato or with salad.

ANTI-CANDIDA DIET

☺ **BREAKFASTS:** home-made muesli with oatflakes and other whole grains mixed with seeds, soaked in water and eaten with soya milk, Rice Dream or natural yoghurt; Shredded Wheat with Rice Dream; puffed oats, puffed wheat or puffed rice with soya milk or Rice Dream; porridge made with water or soya milk, sprinkled with cinnamon or nutmeg and eaten with yoghurt; egg (boiled, poached or scrambled) eaten with wholewheat soda bread or toast and butter; rice cakes with cottage cheese; slices of tinned peas pudding with tomato, grilled or heated in the microwave - and many more besides!

☺ **MAIN MEALS:** try to find a butcher selling free range chickens, also 'organic' lean meat to avoid hormones and antibiotics, (lamb and rabbit are less likely to be affected), but don't forget that red meat has inflammatory properties. Enjoy any type of fish, but oily fish is particularly beneficial (herrings, sardines, mackerel, salmon, tuna). Combine a cereal with a pulse for a complete vegetarian protein, e.g., bean and vegetable pie or crumble, rice or bulgar with chickpeas in a tomato or soya milk and herb sauce, whole wheat spaghetti with brown lentils, tomatoes and onions.

☺ **FRESH VEGETABLES** of all types, steamed. Aim to have a plateful of SALAD every day.

☺ **AVOCADOS** are good filled with cottage cheese and hummus, or yoghurt with tomato puree, topped with slices of cucumber.

☺ **LEMONS;** if adding a slice to your drinks, first scrub the peel well to remove traces of mould. Use lemon juice for salad dressing, for a yoghurt sauce with casseroled chicken and for squeezing over fish.

☺ **SEEDS AND FRESHLY CRACKED NUTS** make nutritious snacks. (Nuts out of their shells have unseen mould.)

☺ **HERBS** of all kinds, fresh or dried, add interesting variations in flavour to your meals.

☺ **MILD SPICES** also add interest (cinnamon, coriander, cumin, turmeric, etc.) but avoid all hot spices and curries because of their effect on the friendly bacteria in your intestines.

☺ **HOT DRINKS:** Barleycup and any type of herb tea or fruit tea provided it has no added citric acid or malt. Rooibosch tastes closest to 'ordinary' tea. Hot tomato juice makes a nice winter warmer!

☺ **COLD DRINKS:** mineral water, still or sparkling, with added ice and lemon not only looks good but is refreshing and delicious. Chilled tomato juice is good as a 'starter', and iced fruit teas (no citric acid or malt!) make a tasty alternative to fruit juice in summer. Try whisking yoghurt with sparkling mineral water and added mint or vanilla essence!

THREE DAYS' SAMPLE MENUS
from the
BEAT CANDIDA COOKBOOK

(All recipes are given in the following section)

DAY 1

Breakfast
Porridge

Lunch
Home-made baked beans with soda bread and salad

Dinner
Tomato and tuna topping with wholewheat spaghetti or instant wholewheat noodles. Sliced green beans, fresh or frozen

Dessert
Yoghurt surprise

DAY 2

Breakfast
Muesli base with soya milk or natural yoghurt

Lunch
Hummus with oatcakes and crudites

Dinner
Piperade with veggie pile and new potatoes

Dessert
Creamy carob

DAY 3

Breakfast
Fish cakes

Lunch
Pizza scones with salad

Dinner
Bean and vegetable stew with brown rice

Dessert
Lemon cheesecake

RECIPES FOR THE THREE DAYS' MENUS

All the recipes are taken from the BEAT CANDIDA COOKBOOK and have a star rating to denote their simplicity or, put another way, the energy required to prepare them! For recipes requiring the least energy, the rating is one star (*). Basic baking and recipes using a moderate amount of energy have two stars (**). Meals in the Cookbook which could be served for dinner parties and take a fair amount of preparation have three stars (***), but none are included here because many of the * and ** recipes are quite delicious, and there is no point in expending unnecessary energy!

For people with specific food intolerances, e.g. wheat or even all the gluten grains, the Cookbook includes special sections giving advice and additional recipes, although many recipes throughout the book indicate that they are gluten-free.

BREAKFASTS

* OATMEAL PORRIDGE
(Microwave version)
1 cup porridge oats
2 cups water or soya milk or half and half
Optional: pinch of Lo-Salt

Cook, uncovered, on full power for 1-2 minutes, stirring halfway. My own favourite version of this is made with jumbo oats and soya milk, using level measures of each. This makes it really thick and creamy. Topped with a sprinkling of cinnamon, it's quite delicious!

It's almost as easy to make porridge in a saucepan, but you're left with a sticky pan to clean. Make sure you fill it with water as soon as you've poured the porridge!

* OATMEAL PORRIDGE
(Saucepan version)
Ingredients as for microwave verson. Heat in a saucepan, stirring all the time, and boil for one minute.

* MUESLI BASE
1 lb / 450g jumbo oats
12oz/ 350g wheat flakes
12oz/ 350g barley flakes
12oz/ 350g rye flakes

Try throwing in a handful of any seeds you fancy, sunflower, sesame, pumpkin or linseeds. Keep it all in an airtight container. This can also form the basis for:

** CRUNCHY BREAKFAST CEREAL
12oz/ 350g muesli base
2oz/ 50g wheatgerm
2oz/ 50g sunflower seeds
2oz/ 50g sesame seeds
2oz/ 50g desiccated coconut
4-5 tbsp cold pressed olive oil

Heat the oven to 350° F/180°C/Gas 4. Mix together all the ingredients and spread on a large baking sheet. Bake for 45 minutes, stirring every 10-15 minutes. Tip into another flat dish to cool before storing in an airtight container. Serve with natural yoghurt, or with hot or cold soya milk or Rice Dream.

* **FISH CAKES** (serves 1-2, gluten-free)
(Good hot or cold for any meal!)
1 tin pilchards in brine
1 tbsp tomato puree (no citric acid)
1 small onion, finely chopped
1 tsp mixed herbs
1/2 mug soya flour

Mash fish and combine well with all ingredients. Make into burger shapes - 4 large or 6 medium. Grill for 5 minutes each side, or fry in a little olive oil, turning after a few minutes, or bake in preheated oven at 400°F/200°C/Gas 6 for 30 minutes. May be frozen cooked or uncooked.

LUNCHES

* **QUICK HOME-MADE BAKED BEANS** (gluten-free)
2 onions
1 tbsp olive oil
14oz/400g tin tomatoes (no citric acid)
2 tbsp tomato puree (no citric acid)
1 tsp mixed herbs and 1 tsp paprika
freshly-ground black pepper
1 tin haricot beans in salt water (sugar-free)

Finely chop the onions and soften in oil over gentle heat. Add tomatoes, tomato puree, herbs, paprika and pepper. Stir well, mashing tomatoes, and simmer for a few minutes to obtain a fairly thick sauce. It may be put through a blender to make it smooth. Drain and rinse the beans and add to the sauce. Heat through, and serve in a baked potato or on toasted soda bread (recipe below). Can be eaten cold with salad.

** YOGHURT SODA BREAD

1 lb/ ½kg wholewheat plain flour
2 tsps baking powder or sodium or potassium bicarbonate
½pt/300ml natural yoghurt
¼pt/150ml warm water

This will make two small loaves or one large one. If you want to make a batch for the freezer, a 1.5kg bag of flour and a 1 litre tub of yoghurt (with 6 tsps baking powder and ¾ pint/ ½ litre warm water) makes six small loaves. Preheat the oven to 400°F/200°C/Gas 6. Sift the flour and mix in the raising agent, then stir in the yoghurt and warm water. Mix together well then coat the mixture with more flour and well-flour your working surface. No kneading is necessary. If making small loaves, divide into two and make into fairly flat, oval shapes. Cut a cross on the top. Place on a floured tray and bake in a preheated oven for 30 minutes, then turn oven down to 350°F/180°C/Gas 4 for another 20 minutes. To test if it's ready, tap the bottom of the loaf and it should sound hollow. Leave to cool on a wire rack. Six loaves in the oven might require a little longer baking. (Beware of fan-assisted ovens with this recipe; it doesn't seem to work!)

* HUMMUS (gluten-free)

1 can chick peas (no sugar), rinsed to remove salt
½ - 1 tsp garlic granules according to preference
¼ pt/150ml natural low-fat yoghurt
½ lemon, squeezed

Mix all ingredients in food processor or blender; leave slightly lumpy. Keep refrigerated.

** OATCAKES (wheat-free)

5oz/150g medium oatmeal
1 tsp unsalted butter
4 fl oz/125ml boiling water

Preheat oven to 350°F/180°C/Gas 4. Put oatmeal into a bowl. Put butter into a heatproof jug and pour the boiling water onto it. When the butter has melted, pour liquid onto the oatmeal and mix well. Leave for a few minutes till oatmeal swells and becomes workable. Turn on to well-floured board and divide into two balls. Roll each ball into a small round and cut across it four times to make eight wedges. Roll each wedge very thinly. Place on baking sheet and bake for about 30 minutes. Wedges will be slightly curved and light golden.

* CRUDITES

Many raw vegetables are suitable, e.g. carrots, celery, cucumber, cauliflower, peppers, radishes, swedes, mooli (long white radishes). You can cut some into matchsticks, some into rings or slices, and cauliflower of course makes pretty florets. Choose three or four with contrasting colours and use a variety of shapes.

** PIZZA SCONES

Base:
8oz/225g plain wholemeal flour
2 tsps baking powder
2oz/50g unsalted butter
4 fl oz/125ml soya milk
Topping:
14oz/400g tin tomatoes (no citric acid)
1 medium chopped onion
1 tbsp cold-pressed olive oil
1/2 tsp mixed herbs or oregano
Extra topping ideas: prawns, tuna, cottage cheese, sweetcorn, green pepper, cooked chicken, etc.

Preheat oven to 425°F/220°C/Gas 7. Sift dry ingredients, rub in butter. Add soya milk and mix to a soft dough. Knead lightly on floured surface, roll out to 1/2 inch/12 mm thickness. Cut out 2 1/2 in./5cm rounds and place on floured baking sheet. Bake for 10-12 minutes. While scones are baking, heat the oil in a pan, add the onions and cook gently until soft. Chop the tomatoes and add to pan together with herbs, and cook till sauce is reduced to jam-like consistency. Remove scones from oven, cut in halves and put them back on the baking sheet, cut side up. Put a spoonful of mixture on each and spread it to the edges. Put on any extra toppings, then bake for a further 10-12 minutes.

DINNERS

* TOMATO AND TUNA TOPPING (gluten-free)

1 dsp tomato puree (no citric acid)
1/4 pt/150ml water
1 small chopped onion
1 small tin tuna in brine (rinsed)
pinch of oregano

Mix tomato puree with the water, add onion and cook over low heat for a few minutes until onion is soft. Flake the tuna and add it with oregano to the pan. Cook until heated through and liquid has reduced a little. Serve with soda bread toast, baked potato or wholewheat pasta.

* PIPERADE (serves 2-4, gluten-free)

1 medium onion, finely chopped
2 cloves garlic, crushed (or 1tsp garlic granules)
2 tbsp cold-pressed olive oil
2 green or red peppers or mixed, seeded and chopped
4 tomatoes, roughly chopped
6 eggs
fresh parsley, finely chopped

Soften the onion and garlic in the oil over a gentle heat for 5 minutes, then add the peppers and tomatoes for a further 5 minutes. Beat the eggs in a separate bowl, then pour over the cooked vegetables and mix them in until lightly scrambled. Garnish with parsley. Cut into required number of servings.

* **VEGGIE PILE** (gluten-free)
8 sticks of celery, chopped
1 large green pepper, seeded and sliced long
1 large red or yellow pepper, seeded and sliced
2 large courgettes, sliced into rounds
Alternatives: sliced white cabbage, broccoli, etc.

Put all vegetables into a large saucepan or wok with a lid, with just a puddle of boiling water in the bottom. Boil fast for no more than four minutes, but take off the lid and stir a few times during cooking. If you need a nutritious fill-up just for yourself, divide the quantities by four and use a small saucepan.

* **BEAN AND VEGETABLE STEW**
2 tins of kidney or haricot beans or chick peas (no sugar)
2 medium onions, chopped
1 green pepper, seeded and chopped
4 large cups of any other vegetables, chopped
water to cover
2 tbsp fine oatmeal mixed with 8 tbsp cold water
4 tbsp tomato puree (no citric acid)
1 tsp dried mixed herbs

Lightly cook the vegetables in water which just covers them. When tender, mix the oatflour and water in a bowl, then add some of the hot vegetable juice to it, stirring carefully. When the paste is smooth, add it to the hot water with the vegetables, stirring all the time. Cook for two minutes, till the gravy is thick, then stir in the tomato puree and herbs. Lastly, drain and thoroughly rinse the beans, then tip them in with the vegetables and heat through gently, making sure that the gravy doesn't 'catch' on the bottom. Serve with wholegrain rice. (Alternatively, and with very little more effort, this can have a crumble topping made from oats and sunflower or olive oil, and baked for 25-30 minutes.)

DESSERTS

* YOGHURT SURPRISE
Mix together:
1 small tub natural yoghurt
1 tbsp pumpkin seeds
1 tbsp sunflower seeds
1 tbsp linseeds
1 tbsp wheatgerm
Optional: 1 tbsp lecithin granules or 2 tbsp whole puffed rice

** CREAMY CAROB DESSERT
3 x 1½oz/ 42g bars plain carob (Plamil dairy-free, sugar-free)
16 fl oz/ 500ml soya milk
4 drops natural vanilla essence
1 tsp agar-agar
8 tbsp cold water

Break up two carob bars into a basin and stand in a saucepan of hot water. Whilst melting, gently heat the soya milk then gradually pour onto the carob, stirring all the time. Add vanilla essence. When mixed together well, remove from heat. Put agar-agar into the cold water in a saucepan and bring to the boil. When dissolved, allow to cool then stir into the carob mixture. Pour through a sieve into a glass bowl or into individual glasses. Chill in refrigerator until set like blancmange then decorate top with grated carob from the other bar. This mixture can be used as a filling for choux pastry cases and even turned into profiteroles with melted carob on top, in which case it should be blended in a liquidiser just before use to make it creamy rather than set!

** LEMON CHEESECAKE
Base:
1 tbsp unsalted butter
1 egg
4oz/125g wholemeal flour
½ tsp baking powder

Melt butter in a saucepan, beat the egg and add to butter. Sift flour with baking powder, add to saucepan and mix well. Press dough into the bottom of a buttered tin.

Topping:
1 lb/450g cottage cheese
4 eggs, separated
juice of 1/2 lemon

Preheat oven to 350°F/180°C/Gas 4. Mix together the cheese, egg yolks and lemon juice. Whisk the egg whites till stiff, fold into mixture with metal spoon. Pour onto prepared base in tin, bake for 40-45 minutes till slightly brown. Allow to cool. May be chilled in refrigerator or served at room temperature.

AND FOR GOOD MEASURE, HERE'S A CARROT CAKE (**) TO HELP FILL YOU UP!

1 egg
4 tbsp unsalted butter
2 cups grated carrot
1 1/2 cups plain wholemeal flour
1 tsp baking powder
1/2 tsp cinnamon
soya milk to mix

Preheat oven to 300°F/150°C/Gas 3. Beat together egg and butter then fold in the grated carrot. Sift together the dry ingredients and mix in well. Add a little soya milk if the mixture seems dry. Pour into loaf tin brushed with olive oil or melted butter, and bake for 1 hour. Allow to stand a little, then turn out carefully onto wire rack to cool.

Now it only remains for me to wish you well as you start to eat your way to health. I hope you enjoy the recipes!

How to learn more about Nutrition

The Institute for Optimum Nutrition runs the following courses:
Homestudy Course (Seventy hours)
Nutrition Consultants Diploma Course (Three years)
Optimum Nutrition Workshop (One day)
Advanced Nutrition Intensive (Six days)
Optimum Nutrition Education (One year)

For further information and news of Open Days and Conferences, contact:
I.O.N., Blades Court, Deodar Road, London SW15 2NU
Telephone 0181 877 9993

Also contact I.O.N. for help in finding other qualified Nutritionists.

Action for M.E. may be contacted at P.O. Box 1302, Wells, BA5 2WE.

The Author may be contacted through the Publishers:

White Publications, 22 Leigh Hall Road, Leigh-on-Sea,
Essex SS9 1RN Telephone 01702 72085

Erica White is available for personal or postal nutritional consultations. All clients receive detailed questionnaires from which their nutritional status and candida potential is assessed. They receive a full printed report with findings and recommendations together with an explanatory covering letter or a personal consultation. This is followed by three months of "back-up" within the price of the consultation to enable ongoing support. A review analysis is recommended after three months. Fees on request.